cancer slam

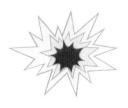

cancer slam

ansley m. dauenhauer

Three Towers Press

milwaukee, wisconsin

Published by
Three Towers Press
A Division of HenschelHAUS Publishing, Inc.
2625 S. Greeley Street, Suite 201
Milwaukee, WI 53207
www.HenschelHAUSbooks.com

Please contact the publisher for quantity discounts.

ISBN: 978-159598-133-2

Library of Congress Cataloging Number: 2011931263

Publisher's Cataloging-In-Publication Data
(Prepared by The Donohue Group, Inc.)

Dauenhauer, Ansley M.
Cancer slam / Ansley M. Dauenhauer.
p. ; cm.
Summary: After her mother is diagnosed with breast cancer, Hannah discovers that
life goes on, even in the face of adversity. She learns a lot about breast cancer and a bit
about herself, too.
Interest age group: 009-013.
ISBN: 978-1-59598-133-2
1. Children of cancer patients--Juvenile fiction. 2. Children of cancer patients--
Psychology--Juvenile fiction. 3. Breast--Cancer--Patients--Family relationships--
Juvenile fiction. 4. Breast--Cancer--Fiction. I. Title.

PZ7.D28 Can 2012
[Fic]   2011931263

Cover design by EM Graphics, Madison, WI

Author photo by Lisa Weldy.

Printed in the United States of America.
2nd printing

For Maddie and Joseph,
the inspiration for Hannah and Max,

and for Mark,
who is everything to me.

table of contents

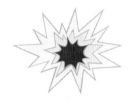

foreword

a new diagnosis of breast cancer is not only frightening for the woman who has the diagnosis, but also for her family. In my two decades of experience treating women with this disease, I have noticed that the children of patients with breast cancer can often have an unrealistic, distorted, and typically unnecessarily dark sense of what the diagnosis means and what the treatments involve. The availability of easily digestible resources for parents and children to demystify and clarify the diagnosis, its implications, and the impact of surgery, drug therapy, and radiotherapy is uneven at best.

In her first novel, *Cancer Slam*, Ansley Dauenhauer offers a thoughtful, story-based lesson for parents with breast cancer to share with their children. The characters are credible, and the experience and dialogue resonate with realism, no doubt based on the author's own personal experience with breast cancer. There are plenty of moments for grinning, smiling, and even laughing through the story of this family as they navigate their experience of breast cancer. The humor helps the medicine go down, so to speak.

I recommend this novel as a very welcome and needed way to help children aged 8 to 12 who often imagine a much more frightening and pessimistic picture of what Mom is facing than the reality may dictate. It can certainly serve as a platform for discussions that will hopefully lead to a more restful night's sleep for both parents and children alike.

Dr. Andrew Seidman
Medical Oncologist and
Attending Physician,
Breast Cancer Medicine Service
Memorial Sloan-Kettering Cancer Center
New York City, NY

x

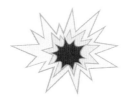

author's note

the first thing I did when I was diagnosed with breast cancer was look for books to read to my children. We found a number of wonderful picture books for the preschool-aged set, but my middle-grade daughter needed something more. In addition to the facts about breast cancer, she needed a story that encompassed all aspects of the life of a child who had lived through breast cancer.

Though breast cancer is, in some ways, a collection of facts, having cancer in the family is an event fraught with emotion. Somehow life goes on, even after your mom has been diagnosed, had surgery, and is in chemotherapy. My daughter had to navigate the waters of telling her friends, as well as dealing with those who already knew. She had to cope with a suddenly bald mom when the last thing she wanted was for either of us to stand out. And she had to figure out how to keep her life going when sometimes nothing seemed to be "going" at home—those were the days Mom crawled in bed and didn't budge.

We were blessed. We had lots of wonderful friends and family who stepped in and helped us out. We didn't have to cook for months. Even so, there are some things you just have to deal with yourself, and a cancer diagnosis will almost certainly force you to find and face those things. Sometimes, though, it's good to have a little help in the facing, even if it's just the knowledge that other people have dealt with cancer too.

In *Cancer Slam*, I took our family's experience with breast cancer and fictionalized it—sometimes a little, and sometimes a lot. Regardless, I hope that after reading this book, you will understand more about the facts of breast cancer and also, maybe even more importantly, see that life does keep going. In some ways things change, but in other ways it's the same. Hannah's brother Max doesn't stop annoying her even on the day they learn about Mom's cancer. But he also doesn't stop loving her, and she can't help loving him back. It's also OK, and often very good, to laugh as much as you can through the tough times. It's even better to talk about what you are feeling, even if what you feel seems wrong. You are almost certainly not the only person to feel that way.

Visit me at www.ansleymdauenhauer.com. There are some links to resources we found helpful for dealing with breast cancer. You will also find some pictures of the "real" Hannah and Max, my children Maddie and Joseph. In the meantime, enjoy getting to know Hannah and Max!

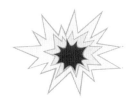

chapter 1
the boo-boo

"**m**aybe," Hannah muttered to herself, "I can hypnotize myself with Lydia's ponytail." Mesmerized by the rhythmic swishing in front of her, Hannah wiped September sweat off her forehead. She wished again that she hadn't cut her hair over the summer. As the lunch-line chatter crackled into background static, there was one thought Hannah couldn't shake: her mom had cancer.

Yesterday, Hannah would have been honored just to be standing behind the owner of those swishing blonde locks. When Lydia had waved her over at lunch, Hannah's smile had nearly burst through her cheeks. Hannah had swooned when Lydia leaned over her lunch, that luxurious hair shielding the two of them from the rest of the class. When Lydia offered her some fig bars, it didn't matter that Hannah hated fig bars; Hannah couldn't believe she was the chosen one. Then the sun had been shining. Hannah couldn't wait for recess.

Today, she hoped it would rain. A rainy recess meant a movie in the auditorium. She wouldn't have to talk to anyone. Maybe, Hannah thought, it will rain for the entire year.

Yesterday, she'd worried whether Ms. Calde was going to bring up the history project.

Today, she was worried that her mom might die.

Hannah ran her fingers through her sweaty bangs. How could she not have paid attention to the bandage peeking out from Mom's shirt that afternoon a few weeks ago?

"It's just a boo-boo," Mom had assured Max, Hannah's four-year-old brother, as he fingered the bandage's ragged edge. Hannah had rolled her eyes—it was so weird for grown-ups to talk about having boo-boos. Mom had continued, "The doctor took a little bit out to see if it is infected."

That was shrugged off easily enough. A little magic cream (what Max called antibiotic ointment) and a bandage, and—hey, presto!—cured boo-boo. Even Hannah, the master worrier, hadn't been worried.

But this wasn't any old boo-boo. The new books on the sofa had been the tip-off. Every one of them featured the word *cancer* somewhere in the title, and one even mentioned a boo-boo. Hannah's chest had tightened. Could Mom's boo-boo be cancer?

Then Hannah had gotten mad. Cancer was *not* a boo-boo. A boo-boo was scraping your knee at the park. A boo-boo was a scratch on your nose from falling off your bike. A boo-boo was a paper cut. Cancer was not, in any way, shape, or form, a boo-boo. Pretending it was, well, that was a lie.

Cancer was being really sick. Cancer meant you could die. You could not fix cancer with magic cream and a Band-Aid. Exactly how old did her parents think she was? Hannah felt duped, and the master-worrier side of her went into high gear.

2

Just then, Maximilian Douglas (Max or M.D. for short) had taken a running leap and landed on the coffee table. He knocked Hannah down and tumbled over on to the pile of books. Max couldn't read yet, so he didn't know what was coming. For a minute, Hannah wished she could be four again.

As Mom sat down on the sofa and Max snuggled into the crook of her arm, Hannah had picked herself up from the floor. Mom raised her other arm to let Hannah in, but instead Hannah just shrugged. "I'd rather go to my room." On her way out of the living room, Hannah had stopped long enough to snap over her shoulder, "I'm really too old to be read to."

"Does Mom think she can just read to us and it will all be OK?" Hannah muttered angrily to herself.

Hannah watched as Max snuggled deeper into Mom's chest. Mom ruffled his hair—the back of his strawberry-colored hair stood up no matter what Mom did to plaster it down. This afternoon, though, Mom didn't fight Max's Mohawk hair-do. She just stroked it in all its spiky glory.

Hannah really wanted to put her head on Mom's chest, too. She loved it when Mom smoothed her hair, which was longer and thicker (and a more mousy-brown) than M.D.'s. Resolutely, Hannah resumed her march down the hall to the room she shared with her brother.

Sometimes Hannah wished her family didn't live in New York City. If they lived in a house, then she could have her own bedroom. Planning for her 'someday' room was one of her favorite past-times. The color scheme was always turquoise with a white bed, but the most important feature was a door to keep out annoying little brothers. No cars, trucks, or motorized vehicles would be allowed anywhere in her territory.

Hannah stepped over the toy cars Max had abandoned in that morning's rush, climbed the bunk bed ladder, and threw herself down on her mattress. She closed her eyes, ready to envision her future sanctuary. But instead of pastel walls, all she saw were those books on the sofa screaming, "Cancer! Cancer! Your mom has cancer!"

Hannah flipped over to face her special shelf, where she kept her prized possessions high above Max's clumsy fingers. The sea glass she had found last summer in Maine was cradled in a bath of soft gray shadows. The orange flush of the late afternoon sun lit the wall behind it. Hannah squeezed her eyes shut, willing the wind from the Maine ocean to blow through the windows. Instead, giggles floated in from the living room.

What could be so funny? There was certainly nothing funny about cancer. But still, everything had been so somber the past few days that Hannah realized she'd missed laughing.

She glared at the ceiling a few more minutes before sighing and hauling herself down the ladder. Grabbing a tattered book from the shelf, Hannah crept out to the living room to read.

Mom's fingers drummed softly on the cover of one of the unopened books in her lap as she listened to Max's chatter.

His eyes stared at a map of the world hanging on the wall. "Mommy, what side of the world are we on?" Max asked.

"We live in the Western Hemisphere," Mom replied.

"No, I mean are we on the upside or the downside?"

Mom groaned softly while Max tilted his head so that it was parallel to the equator.

Mom followed Max's gaze to the map on the wall. "On that map," Mom pointed to the United States, which was

4

featured prominently in the center, "we're in the middle. That map is made in the U.S.

"But," Mom twisted around to point to a different map above the sofa, "on this map, we're over here, on the left side. This map is made in China, so China is in the middle. See the characters on top, the Chinese writing?"

"Why do Chinese people think we're in a different place, Mommy?" Max asked.

Mom reached over and flicked on a lamp by Hannah's chair. Hannah glanced down, surprised. She liked to read in the leather chair on the other side of the living room. It was worn and soft with a lamp that arched over it, making it perfect for reading. Today, though, she was sitting in the chair next to the sofa.

With Mom's attention temporarily diverted, Max leaned over, flattened his belly to the sofa, and then threw himself backward onto Mom's outstretched arm. The sofa cushions bounced him forward again, making him laugh hysterically. Through his giggles, he demanded, "Mommy, why do we live in the Western 'mimispere? Why, Mommy? Why? I want to know!"

Mom shot Max a gently exasperated look. "Dad's job is in the Western Hemisphere, our apartment is in the Western Hemisphere, and your school is in the Western Hemisphere. So we live in the Western Hemisphere."

Mom took a deep breath and eyed Max firmly before continuing. "Sometimes the Western Hemisphere is shown on the right side of the map and sometimes it's shown on the left side. It just depends. If the map is made in the U.S., then the U.S. is in the center. If it's made in China, then China's in the center. The map changes, but the actual location of the people stays the same."

Max opened his mouth, but Mom silenced him. "Where we live is just where God has put us," she said in her no-nonsense voice. When Mom didn't have any more answers for Max, she let God step in. Mom figured even Max couldn't argue with God.

Then Mom had gently grabbed at Max's thigh and worked her fingers into the chunky part just above his knee.

"Mommy, stop! Mommy, stop! That's my tickle spot!" Max had shrieked happily. When Mom pulled her hands back, he had gasped through his giggles, "More, more!" Even in her current black mood, Hannah had had to smile. Max was the only kid in the whole world who liked being tickled.

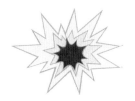

chapter 2
ronald mcdonald

that was yesterday. Now, Hannah followed Lydia's ponytail down the hall and into the lunchroom. The perfect swish had slowed to an irregular bounce. Hannah's hypnosis attempt wasn't working anyway. She sighed. Cancer, cancer, cancer! Everything screamed cancer.

Hannah sniffed as they lined up for hot lunch. Hamburgers and French fries. Then she rubbed her forehead wearily. It really was a conspiracy. Cancer *was* everywhere. "French fries can't cure cancer," Hannah muttered under her breath.

"Maybe not," Scottie broke through her haze, "but they sure taste better than some of the other cafeteria offerings."

"Huh?" Hannah turned and then blushed. She'd been talking out loud.

"Since when does anyone think French fries could cure cancer?" Scottie ribbed her.

Ignoring him, Hannah claimed her tray. If only French fries *could* cure cancer, she thought wistfully, she'd be happy to share a room with Ronald McDonald *and* her brother.

Hannah smiled a little remembering Max's giggle-fest yesterday afternoon. When he finally stopped laughing, Mom had asked if they knew what cancer was. Max shook his head, but Hannah had stayed very still, hoping if she didn't move, the word would just evaporate. It didn't. Instead, it weighed down the whole room. Even Max felt the pressure, because he stopped wiggling and stayed very close to Mom.

The books had slipped off Mom's lap and were loose on the sofa. Hannah thought that Mom probably didn't want to read them any more than Hannah wanted to hear them. Finally Mom picked up the one on top and read it out loud.

At the end, Mom took a deep breath and said, "The 'boo-boo' in my breast is cancer." The word was out, circling so fast it blurred, dive-bombing its poison into their living room and into their lives.

Cancer…so the boo-boo *was* cancer. In the ensuing fog, Hannah replayed the past few weeks. All she could recall was school-related stuff—meeting Lydia and shyly asking her to play at recess, joking with Scottie, her buddy from Pre-K, and praying that she would be one of the kids on Ms. Calde's good side.

When had Mom found the lump? When did she and Dad find out it was cancer? And, the essence of it all, would Mom die?

Everyone talked about fighting cancer. But, a fight meant there were winners and losers. If you lose the cancer fight, does that mean you die? Hannah cringed. Could her mom be a loser? How do you fight cancer anyway? Cancer wasn't a thing. As much as Hannah wanted to, she couldn't hit it. The word oozed through her brain, an amorphous blob leisurely lacing its tentacles in and around everything. Hannah laid her head on the back of the chair and closed her eyes. Couldn't it just go away?

Max sat straight up and immediately asked, "Will you get to live at Ronald McDonald's house?"

Mom's forehead scrunched into a question mark. "Why would I go there?" she asked, rubbing circles on Max's back with her fingertips.

"Because that's where Rose lived," Max explained, nodding excitedly.

"Rose?" Both Mom and Hannah looked at Max, perplexed. "Who is Rose?"

"Rose, that girl in Hannah's class last year. She had canker. She got to live with Ronald McDonald at his house."

"Oh, Rose," Mom said, nodding with understanding. Then Mom brightened and gestured towards the window. "No! Look how lucky we are. We live ten blocks from one of the best cancer hospitals in the world. I get to stay right here at home."

"You don't want to live with Ronald McDonald?" Max asked, puzzled.

"Rose's home was a long way from New York, " Mom explained. "She needed to see doctors here. That's why she and her mom had to live at the Ronald McDonald House while she got treatment for her cancer. We already live near a cancer center. I don't have to go anywhere."

Hannah felt a small wave of relief. She looked around the apartment, appreciating the bright yellow of the walls. It was Mom's favorite color. Hannah was so relieved Mom didn't have to go away, not just from the apartment, but from them, from her, Max, and Dad.

Max asked, "Even if you don't get to live with Ronald, will you still get to eat lots of French fries? And, Mommy," Max added hopefully, "will you please share them with us?"

"What are you talking about?!" Hannah exploded. "French fries? Mom has cancer. Let's not give her a cholesterol problem, too!" Her class was studying food and its effect on the human body, and Mom having more than one health problem was more than Hannah could bear.

Max's eyes shrunk to small slits, a sure sign he was about to cry.

"French fries at Ronald McDonald's house!" Max choked out. "We get French fries when we see Ronald McDonald at his rest'rant, so he prob'ly has them at his house, too."

Mom intervened with a small smile and a squeeze for Max. "Ronald McDonald doesn't actually live at the Ronald McDonald House," she explained. "The same company that started McDonald's restaurants gave money to set up the Ronald McDonald Houses. That's why they have the same name. Ronald McDonald Houses are special places where moms and dads whose children are in the hospital can stay. Sometimes they have to stay there many months."

Mom shook her head slowly, continuing, "I don't know if they serve French fries, though. I think people mostly do their own cooking while they live there."

Max sniffed indignantly, "Well, they should give the sick people French fries. It would make them feel better."

Mom grinned and agreed, "Yum! I love hot, salty French fries. They would definitely make me feel better."

"Do you feel bad right now?" Max worried, snuggling closer to her.

Mom smiled down at him and shook her head. "No. It's kind of crazy, isn't it? I have this disease, but I don't feel bad. But the things that will get me well are going to make me feel lousy." She glanced around the apartment with a small sigh.

Hannah had followed Mom's gaze. For the first time since they'd gotten home, Hannah noticed the toys and books strewn everywhere.

"Maybe," Hannah had thought, "maybe I should try to be a little better at picking up stuff. Just for her. At least for now."

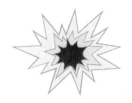

chapter 3
cancer—day 2

h annah slid her tray between Scottie's and Lydia's at the lunch table. She poked unenthusiastically at the limp potatoes. At least McDonald's fries aren't soggy, even if they can't cure cancer, she thought.

Not only was cancer suddenly everywhere, but it was affecting everything, too.

This morning when she had woken up, the feeling of dread was heavier than just the usual time-to-get-up dismay. Then Hannah remembered the afternoon before and the fact that Mom had cancer. Suddenly she thought about the upcoming camping trip. It was their first one and so many cousins from both sides of their family, Jenny and Liam, Aunt Kath and Uncle Jeff, Will, Hugh, and Jimmy, were coming. It was sure to be a real party. "Oh no," Hannah had moaned from under the covers.

Mom, who was on the floor trying to wrestle Max into his school clothes, looked up at the top bunk from the floor with raised eyebrows.

"Don't tell me we're going to have to miss the camping trip because of your operation!" Hannah groaned.

Mom managed to jerk Max's trousers on before he flopped onto the floor. Mom rocked back on her heels, reached for his socks, and gazed up at Hannah, who was still an immobile lump under the covers.

"Well," Mom said, a hint of understanding woven into her voice, "we are going to try very hard to make the camping trip happen, but I can't promise anything."

Hannah sighed. Mom and Dad were always very careful not to make unkeepable promises. The good part of that was that when they did make a promise, Hannah could count on it. The bad part was that they didn't actually promise all that much. If Mom wasn't promising, there was a very real possibility the camping trip wasn't happening.

Just then Max sighed, too. Looking at his fully-socked feet, Max conceded victory, "Oh, Mommy, you just captured my toes." Mom patted him consolingly on the bum and told him to make up his bed.

Next Mom turned her attention to Hannah. "Come on, Sleepyhead," she said, trying to prod Hannah from her nest. Hannah burrowed deeper under the covers. Hannah hated mornings, and she really hated how Max always woke up chipper and ready to go.

About that time, Dad strode into the room, all showered and smooth from shaving. "Hey, Max-Buddy! Good bed-making!" Dad announced cheerfully and then put the full-court press on Hannah.

"Where's my Hannah-Banana? Good morning! Time to get up and get ready for another big day!"

13

Mom promptly headed into the kitchen to make breakfast, leaving Dad with the problem of getting Hannah out of bed.

Dad flew Hannah off the top bunk, a private joke they shared from nursery school. She kept her long legs very stiff to keep from kicking Dad while he zoomed her out of the room. Max followed along, chattering incessantly about the camping trip. Suddenly Max decided Dad needed to get the sleeping bags out *right now*. (Hannah often thought Max's middle name should have been Impatience, instead of Douglas.)

Mom stuck her head into the hall and interrupted Max to ask what he wanted for breakfast. Max fell over shrieking that he couldn't eat breakfast until his sleeping bag was out. Hannah looked down at him from her perch in Dad's arms and crossed her eyes. Mom rubbed her forehead wearily. Dad lowered Hannah carefully to the floor, his eyebrows raised at Max. The three of them exchanged glances and started laughing.

Max bristled indignantly. It was one of those mornings when he wasn't getting the respect he felt he deserved. He squinted up at them, ready to scream some more when he saw Hannah's crossed eyes. Then he giggled, crossed his own eyes, and stood up. Mom turned back to the kitchen, shaking her head, and Dad sent M.D to the table and Hannah to the bathroom.

Most families try to eat dinner together, but the Bennetts almost always ate breakfast together instead. Dad had to work late most evenings, so Mom usually ate with Hannah and Max. But all four of them were at the table almost every morning, discussing the day ahead or upcoming family events.

This morning, the topic was camping. Dad shot Mom a look across the table. Mom gave him a tight smile. "I told Hannah we couldn't promise, but we would really try."

Max chimed in, "Because of your canker."

"Cancer! Not canker," Hannah snapped. Not only could Max not say the word, but he didn't even sound worried, about Mom or the camping trip.

Dad said, "We just don't know yet when Mom's operation will be."

Suddenly Hannah thought of all the things that happen in October—her birthday being one of the more important events. They could cancel camping if they had to, but they couldn't cancel her birthday, could they? And her birthday party, what would happen to that? No one had mentioned that either, and the date was getting close. That wasn't a good sign.

When Hannah looked around, Max and Dad were discussing the tent situation. Dad really thought they needed a bigger tent and a two-burner cook stove, whatever that was. Hannah looked at Mom. Mom was shaking her head. Clearly she didn't want a two-burner cook stove, but she did think Hannah and Max needed new sleeping bags because the ones they had weren't meant for sleeping outdoors.

Dad thought a minute and then grinned. "Well, I can wrap up in a blanket." Then, pointing to Mom, he continued, "We'll wrap you in your down coat," and waving his hands towards Hannah and Max, he finished, "the two of them can have our sleeping bags. Then everyone will be nice and toasty!"

Mom's laugh was thin. "If I don't get enough sleep...," she warned.

15

Hannah mentally filled in the blank, "you won't be happy, and if you're not happy, we're not happy." Sleep was very important to Mom. So was getting to school on time, and suddenly Mom went into a flurry of activity, handing out lunchboxes, checking for brushed teeth, and rushing everyone out the door, in the hopes of beating the first school bell.

h annah had headed off to school, still in shock that her mom had cancer. Cancer happened to other people. It wasn't supposed to happen to your own family. Besides, Mom was healthy—she made them eat fruit with their snack, they almost always had two vegetables at dinner, and Mom exercised most days. She did all the things Hannah had learned in science that were important for staying well.

Now Hannah looked down the lunch table. Scottie was putting bunny ears on Carl, trying to get some laughs. Carl was attempting, like he did every day, to trade his vegetables for whatever disgusting glop the cafeteria called dessert. Hannah thought suddenly, "Why not Carl's mom?" Not that she wanted Carl's mom to have cancer, but Carl never ate vegetables. His family couldn't be too healthy. So why didn't they get cancer?

Hannah thought about their neighbors in the apartment next door. They only exercised when they wanted to lose weight. Not that they needed to lose weight, Hannah reasoned, but why didn't they get cancer? Why her own family? Why the Bennetts?

At recess, Ellie found her by the wall. "Our class hasn't found out any more about the history project. Have you guys?"

16

"No," Hannah replied shortly. Ellie had been one of her best friends for about forever, but right now Hannah just wanted her to go away.

Ellie looked at her in surprise and tried again, "I signed out a ball today. Do you want to play two-square?"

"No," Hannah repeated, feeling mean as she walked away. She didn't want to talk to anyone. She was afraid she might cry. How embarrassing would that be? Worse, then she'd have to explain why she was crying. For some reason, she didn't want anyone to know about the cancer.

The afternoon droned on until 2:40, time for Sam's birthday celebration. As he passed out his cupcakes, Hannah thought about her own upcoming celebration. And what about Halloween? Thanksgiving? And Christmas, for crying out loud! Those books yesterday talked about how cancer treatment went on for months. Even Christmas, the holiday furthest away, was in just a couple of months. Surely the cancer couldn't stop Christmas from coming?

Hannah allowed herself a small laugh. The master worrier in her was taking over, and she knew she sounded like the Grinch. She reminded herself that even the Grinch, the grinchy ol' Grinch, couldn't stop Christmas from coming. It came. Just like her birthday would, and Halloween, and Thanksgiving, and even Christmas. Cancer couldn't just erase those from the calendar. But it still wasn't a very good day.

Hannah wished again for a rainy day recess, for rain for the rest of the year. But the sun continued to shine, at least for day two of the Cancer Slam.

17

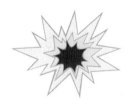

chapter 4
information overload

annah groaned when she came home to more books about somebody's mother getting cancer on the coffee table. Really, how many books about this topic could there possibly be? Besides, did dads ever get cancer? She supposed they couldn't get breast cancer for the obvious reason that they didn't have breasts. (Hannah would learn later that though it's relatively rare, men can get breast cancer. Men do have breast tissue, but it doesn't develop in the same way female breast tissue does. The treatment for men with breast cancer is the same as that for women.) But weren't there other kinds of cancer? Did women who weren't moms ever get breast cancer?

And why was the plot in all of these books always the same? The families started out crying and scared, then the moms would look thin and brave and wear fancy scarves, and finally at the end of the story, everything would be back to normal, except that the moms would have very short hair.

What about all the stuff that happened in the middle? Cancer wasn't all bald heads and fancy scarves, and all of the women didn't get well. Some lost the cancer fight. Her mom could die.

Hannah threw one of the books across the room. The loud clatter it made on the wooden floor did nothing to make her feel better. Her mom could die, and she couldn't picture her family without Mom. Who would take care of them, grocery shop for them, get them where they needed to go? Who would read to them? Who'd tell her when her outfit didn't match, or that her hair needed brushing, or that she'd left the towel on the bathroom floor again? Who would listen when she'd had a bad day at recess? Who would remind her to say her prayers at night?

She couldn't picture herself without Mom. She couldn't picture Dad either—who would make him his dinner and take his suits to the dry cleaners? Who would make sure his sandwiches never had mayonnaise on them? And Max? Who could possibly be patient with Max if Mom wasn't around?

The cancer blob residing in her head stretched its tentacles down to Hannah's lungs and squeezed, making it hard to breathe.

Mom came into the living room. "What was that noise?" she asked. Then Mom noticed the book on the floor. "Hannah, really!" Mom admonished her.

"I know, I know…" Hannah muttered to herself, as Mom picked up the book.

"We respect our books," Mom reminded Hannah, repeating a line she often had to tell Max.

On the first page of one of the new books was a suggestion Max loved. Supposedly cancer would be less scary if they said the word *cancer* one hundred times.

Max immediately jumped off the sofa and hopped in rhythm, "Canker one, canker two…," his chant growing louder with each repetition.

Mom tried to cajole Hannah into counting with them, but Hannah just shook her head. Chant *cancer*? Come on! Repeating the word didn't change its meaning, and shouting it didn't get rid of it either. Every time the word *cancer* was said, Hannah felt it release more of its poison, tightening its grip on them.

Just because every single cancer book ended with everything back to normal, there was no guarantee for the Bennett family. Even Mom, after she had read them the first book, said, "This isn't exactly our story. Let's change the important details." Hannah knew Mom was talking about easy things, like where the characters lived and how old they were. But the ending of the story was a pretty important detail, and Hannah was afraid their ending might be different.

Max stumbled on the numbers and pleaded for help, "Thirty-nine…thirty-ten…Hanny, that's not right. It's not thirty-ten! What is it?" Hannah decided to make an exit for their bedroom.

Just as she stood up, Mom asked, "Do you want to feel the lump?"

Hannah froze as Max instantly put his hands all over Mom's shirt. Mom got hold of his hands and moved them gently to the lump. This time, M.D. just used one hand and felt the lump very carefully.

Finally, Mom told him that was enough. Hannah thought she heard her mutter, "Just like a man," under her breath as

Max settled back down on the sofa next to her. Mom turned to face Hannah and raised her eyebrows.

Hannah shook her head and straightened up. Then she reconsidered.

"Well, maybe...Will it hurt you?" she asked Mom nervously.

Mom lay her own fingers on the lump and shook her head sadly. "No, I wish it hurt. Then I'd have known it was there sooner." As Hannah placed her fingers on top of Mom's, Mom slid her own hand away.

Hannah's knuckles lay against the soft skin of Mom's chest, but a bump, almost like a small marble really, protruded against her fingertips. In the pause before Hannah snatched her hand back, she recognized the lump as the cancer, the thing causing all of this trouble.

Mom adjusted her blouse and picked up another book.

This time Hannah slipped next to Mom on the sofa and snuggled into Mom's chest too, the top of her head tucked under Mom's chin. Mom pulled both Hannah and Max close, and Hannah could feel her swallow hard. Hannah smelled lemon starch on Mom's blouse and saw Max's ginger-colored spikes brush Mom's other cheek. For the moment, Hannah felt safe.

21

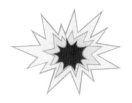

chapter 5
the history project

he dreaded history project reared its ugly head the next day at school. Ms. Calde had divided the class into six groups. Each group was to choose a time period from the ones listed on the board. Each student would then choose an historic site in New York City connected to the group's time period to research. Then each group was to tie the individual research together with an introduction, conclusion, and anything else the group thought would be helpful.

The key, Hannah decided, was going to be in her group. The kids she was going to be working with would make all the difference to this project.

Much groaning went on when Ms. Calde announced the groups, but on the whole, Hannah thought she had been pretty lucky. She and Scottie were known quantities—she knew she would work hard, and as funny as Scottie was, he was also very thoughtful. He really knew when to joke around and when to get down to business. Sam and Mary were the wild cards. Hannah didn't know them yet, but they seemed nice enough; at least they didn't routinely get into trouble.

Hannah's group chose the Revolutionary War. Hannah spent the reading period looking at books Ms. Calde had. Hannah concentrated on the photos, trying to decide which site would be interesting to visit.

On the way to recess, Mary was in front of Hannah. She turned and said quietly, "I'm glad you're in my group. I think it's going to be an interesting project."

"It's a relief to have it out in the open. You know, to know what the project is. The mystery was killing me!" Hannah told her.

Mary agreed, "Yeah, my sister's in junior high, and she had me really scared. She said the teachers always pick a huge project for this year, and they keep it a secret for a few days just to get us scared."

Scottie rushed from behind and poked his head between them. "Do you think we can add some live action to our report? Maybe we can re-enact a battle or something! Or, ride a horse into the class, you know, like Paul Revere!"

"That's Boston, Silly!" Hannah thumped him on the back laughing. "Paul Revere rode through Boston, not New York." Hannah paused a minute, thinking. "Actually, I don't know very much about the Revolutionary War here in New York. All I know about is Boston. My aunt used to live in Boston, so we've been to Lexington and Concord and all of that."

Scottie said, "Well, there had to be a battle around here somewhere. I'm sure we can re-enact something!"

Mary eyed Scottie a little worriedly, but Hannah waved him away dismissively. "Oh don't worry about him. He'll be fine. He's just very enthusiastic!"

23

At pick-up time, Lydia wandered over to where Hannah was waiting in the schoolyard. "I saw you talking with Mary at recess."

"Yeah, she's in my history group. She seems really nice."

"I missed playing with you," Lydia persisted.

Hannah looked surprised. "Well, you should have come over. Mary is super-nice."

"Oh, I was busy playing with the boys," Lydia said , trying to be nonchalant.

"Who's in your history group?" Hannah asked her a bit distractedly while looking around for Mom. It was not unusual for Mom to be a little late, but Hannah hated it when Mom was. Then she and Max had to go to the late table inside the cafeteria. The cafeteria at the end of the day always gave Hannah a headache.

"Carl—he is so cute," Lydia was saying when Hannah felt a hand on her shoulder.

Hannah turned. When she saw the taupe hair and soft wrinkles, she shrieked happily. "Gram! I didn't know you were coming today!" she said excitedly as Gram enfolded her in a huge hug.

"Where's Max?" Hannah asked, looking over Gram's shoulder for her brother.

"I just took Max home. That's why I was a little late. Gramps is there with him."

"But, where's Mom?" Hannah asked nervously.

Gram's eyes filled with tears, which she quickly dabbed away with a tissue. "Your mom had to have some tests before the operation. Gramps and I are here for a day or two so she can see doctors and have whatever else she needs done without worrying about you and your brother."

"Does she know when the operation is yet?" Hannah asked, thinking about the camping trip.

"I don't think so," Gram replied. "Maybe she'll have more information tonight. Should we go home? I know Gramps wants to see you."

Hannah nodded and turned to say goodbye to Ms. Calde. It wasn't until she and Gram were out of the schoolyard that she realized she hadn't said goodbye to Lydia.

"Oh well," Hannah thought, "I'll see her tomorrow."

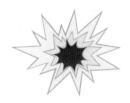

chapter 6
gram, gramps, and a
very long afternoon

annah grabbed Gram's hand as they walked down the block. "I didn't know you were coming today, Gram."

"Well," Gram squeezed Hannah's hand and looked down at her. Gram seemed to be trying to decide what to say.

Finally she started, "When Liz called and told us the news…" Gram pinched her lips together and squeezed her eyes shut before continuing. "Gramps and I wanted to help out any way we could. Today was the quickest we could get organized. We'll stay a day or two for now and then maybe come back for the surgery. Or Papa might come then. Your mom has to figure out what works best for you all. In any case, you're going to see a lot of us for the next few months."

"Well, that's a good surprise!" Hannah returned Gram's squeeze and skipped down the block to their building.

She gave Charlie, their doorman, a high five as she raced to the stairs.

"Oh no," Gram shook her head, calling Hannah back. "I know your parents like to take the stairs, but I take the elevator!"

Hannah grinned, turned her back on the stairway door, and pressed the up button.

When the elevator doors opened on their floor, Hannah started giggling. She could hear the weather channel blasting at full volume all the way down the hall. That would be Gramps. "And I bet he's reading the newspaper, too," Hannah smiled to herself.

Sure enough, when they entered the apartment, Gramps was settled comfortably in the leather chair, his nose buried in the paper. Gram marched over to the television and turned the volume way down.

"Simon! We could hear that all the way down the hall!" Gram fussed.

Hannah slipped under Gram's waving arms and crushed Gramps' newspaper in a big hug.

"Oh," Gramps grunted. Then realizing the source of what had disturbed his reading, he smiled and pulled Hannah to him. "Got any boyfriends yet?" Gramps always asked Hannah about boyfriends.

"Graaammmmmps!" Hannah swatted at him in protest.

"Do that again, this time for me," Gram told her, moving the TV remote away from Gramps' reach.

Max was busy with his trains. Gramps must have helped him put the track together, Hannah thought. It was a particularly complicated one, with lots of turns and bridges. Once Max started in with his trains, he was usually occupied for hours.

Gram offered to let Hannah help make dinner. "I'm going to put a few casseroles together for your freezer. There will probably be some nights your mother won't want to cook," she added.

Hannah hadn't thought of that. She washed her hands and put on an apron. Gram had a cookbook out and was sautéing some vegetables. She handed Hannah some salt and pepper to shake into the frying pan.

"Not too much salt," Gram warned, wiping up some splattered olive oil with a sponge.

Gram busied herself getting the raw meat ready to cook. Then she lifted the baking dish, wiped underneath it, and put it back down on a layer of paper towels. She turned to Hannah.

"Oh, Honey, here, use this damp paper towel to wipe up that salt. Make sure you salt *over* the pan." Gram moved back to the stove and watched closely as Hannah cleaned up the spilled salt.

Hannah stepped away from the stove, bored. She had not inherited her grandmother's ability to clean while she cooked. She sighed. She really missed Mom.

Last week when she and Mom had made biscuits together, the scene had been totally different. "Cut the shortening into the flour," Mom had instructed, demonstrating with a fork. "Hannah, watch that flour. Keep it in the bowl…no, not on the counter, the bowl, use smaller stokes…the flour, you're making a mess! Oh, forget it!"

Then Mom had bent over, like she always did when Hannah cooked, moved the rug from the kitchen floor, and stopped worrying about the mess. When they were done, Mom shooed Hannah from the kitchen so she could clean up.

Even worse than missing Mom was knowing where she was, at the hospital, finding out more information about the cancer.

Hannah took off her apron and slipped out of the kitchen. She picked up her notebook in the living room and started doodling. Lydia had taught her how to make a fairy from a capital "X." Hannah added long hair and a veil. She studied it a moment and decided it looked a little like Cinderella. Then she added the glass slippers and a pretty sash.

Her picture made her think of a Sunday school dress. Of course, a dress wouldn't be nearly as elegant as a ball gown would be, but they did twirl when she spun around, and one had a sash that Mom liked to fuss into a perfect bow. Then Dad would say, "There's my princess."

A princess. That was what she'd said she wanted to be for Halloween at dinner a few weeks ago. She knew some of the kids at school thought they were too old for trick-or-treating, but Hannah loved Halloween and dressing up. She had fun planning out her costume every year. Last year, she'd been a cat in a leotard and tights. The best part of that costume had been the tail. She'd taken one of Dad's belts and fastened it snugly around her waist. The extra belt length hung down the back of her legs, swishing exactly like a tail.

No, Hannah thought, she definitely wasn't ready to give up Halloween yet, but kind of like her birthday party, no one had mentioned Halloween or getting a costume ready recently.

With a last glance at her fairy princess illustration, Hannah abandoned her doodles to check out their dress-up drawer. Maybe there was something in there she could use, just in case Mom and Dad forgot about Halloween altogether. She tugged hard on the drawer. Shoes, purses, hats, scarves, and Max's pirate paraphernalia leapt out and littered the floor. Reaching in, Hannah felt along the drawer seams. She untangled several dresses. Smoothing them out on the bed, she eyed them carefully.

They were a bit faded, and some of the hems were fraying. Worse, they seemed shorter than the last time she'd looked at them. Hannah looked down at her legs. Maybe she'd grown again? It had been quite a while since she played dress up. She looked back at the dresses. A proper princess dress needed to sweep across the floor, preferably over high heels. She would be lucky if these would even cover the bruises on her knees. Hannah already felt like Cinderella, only before her fairy godmother visits.

With nothing to wear for Halloween, Hannah felt the cancer blob stretch its tentacles out of her head and settle heavily into the crevices of the room.

Back in the living room, underneath her picture, Hannah wrote:

"There was a girl whose mother got very sick and she died. 'You have to find someone to take care of us,' she cried to her father. 'Don't worry. I will,' he said."

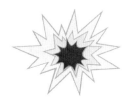

chapter 7
proper princess attire

a couple of mornings later at the breakfast table, Dad commented, "You look pretty tired, Liz." He glanced down at his watch. "I can do school drop-off today. Why don't you take the morning off and rest?"

Alarmed, Hannah looked up at Mom. Dad almost never did school drop-off. Mom's eyes were a little puffy, and she had pulled her hair back like she didn't want to mess with it.

Mom nodded at Dad. "Well, I won't argue with you, if you have time."

As Mom leaned over to give Max a good-bye kiss, she said, "I'll be there to pick you up this afternoon."

"Really?" Max's mouth dropped open. "You? No Gram or Gramps?"

Mom nodded. "Just me. Gram and Gramps left early this morning to visit your aunt. But they'll be back."

"Yippee!" Max shouted, twirling down the hallway. "Hannah! Mommy's going to pick us up today! Nobody else! Just Mommy!"

Hannah smiled. That was good news. Maybe she could pretend things were normal again.

h annah raced into the schoolyard to find Lydia. Lydia hadn't been in school for the past couple of days, and Hannah wanted to apologize. She didn't want Lydia to be mad at her.

Spotting Lydia near their class line, Hannah ran over, puffing, "I'm so sorry I didn't say goodbye the other day. I didn't know my grandmother was going to pick me up, and when I saw Gram, I forgot all about you.

"But look, Lydia," Hannah prattled on. "I've been working on those fairies. We can add all sorts of stuff to them to make them really cool—not just fairies, but princesses, and ballerinas." Hannah held up one of her notebooks.

Lydia stuck her chin in the air and sniffed. "I don't believe you." Lydia was clearly nursing a grudge. "Why would your grandparents surprise you like that? Don't they live far away? I think the truth is that you don't really want to be best friends."

Hannah opened her mouth in surprise, but before she could answer, Mary walked up. "Hi, Hannah!"

Hannah blew out a big gulp of air. Now what was she going to do?

Mary glanced over at the notebook Hannah was holding. "Wow! Those are really cool fairies and princesses. How did you do that?"

Before Hannah could demonstrate, Lydia grabbed the notebook out of her hands and slammed it shut. "That's a secret between Hannah and me."

Mary shrank back, and Hannah looked at Lydia in confusion. "No, it's not," Hannah protested, puzzled.

"Well, it is if you want to keep being best friends," Lydia retorted.

Hannah put out her hands. "Give me back my notebook," she demanded.

Lydia stuck her chin in the air again and thrust the notebook at Hannah. "Fine! If that's the way you want it!" Lydia stalked off towards the group of boys standing near the line.

Hannah shrugged her shoulders. "I don't know what her problem is. But look, Lydia showed me how you make a fairy." She drew a capital X and added a few lines. "Last night I designed all of these others too." Hannah pointed to her princesses and ballerinas.

Mary was impressed. "We could make these into paper dolls," she commented thoughtfully.

With rain at pickup time, dismissal was indoors. Hannah and Mary took advantage of the extra time in the cafeteria to work on their paper doll designs. Mom was right on time that afternoon, but Hannah actually wished she'd been running a little behind.

"'Bye, Mary. I'll try to get a couple of these finished at home tonight."

"Me, too! See you tomorrow!" Mary waved.

Hannah didn't really look at Mom until they were at the corner. When she did, she wasn't sure if it was raindrops or tears that had smeared Mom's mascara, but Mom's eyes were rimmed in black and her cheeks were wet.

Max raced ahead, landing full-throttle in a puddle. With muddy water running down his trouser legs, he laughed like a hyena. Hannah and Mom hurried after him, being careful to dodge his puddle.

By the time they started up the stairs to the apartment, they were all drenched and cold. Mom was definitely not in a good mood, fussing about Max's wet clothes and Hannah's tripping on the stairs. Suddenly, the stair door stopped in mid-creak. Charlie, the building doorman, yelled up at them, "Liz, you have a package!"

Max loved getting packages even when they weren't actually for him. When he heard Charlie's announcement, he yelped in delight and turned on his heels to grab the surprise. Water sprayed out from his soggy shoes and his feet slipped out from under him. He bumped down the stairs on his bum, landing right at Charlie's feet.

For a moment, Mom had looked like she might leave the package for later, but when she saw Max fall, she changed directions and hurried down the stairs to him and his growing puddle.

"Right back up, Buddy!" Mom said, reaching for Max's hands. But looking at his crumpled face, she changed her tactic and sank down beside him on the stairs. "Where do you need a kiss?" Mom asked sympathetically.

Charlie, who was relieved not to have to deal with a hurt Max, waved Hannah back down the stairs too. "Stand here, Princess, and hold the door while I get your package."

"That's all I'm good for," Hannah muttered to herself morosely, "a doorstop."

She put out her arms to take the package from Charlie when he came back, but he held it tight. "This is a heavy one, Hannah. Better let Mommy take it."

Hannah hated when Charlie referred to Mom as Mommy. In the first place, she wasn't his mom. And in the second, Hannah almost never called Mom *Mommy* anymore—only at certain times, like when she was really tired.

However, the arrival of the package did the trick as far as M.D. was concerned. His tears, if not his trousers, dried up immediately, and he couldn't wait to see what it was.

Mom plopped the huge box in the living room floor while they shed everything wet. M.D. was down to his underwear.

"Rebecca," Mom mused, spying the return address label, her black-rimmed eyes actually lighting up a little. "I wonder what she's up to?" Rebecca was Mom's best friend from when she was a little girl, and her son Jake shared the same birthday with Max.

Max got scissors to cut the tape, and Hannah flipped on some lights. The first thing they pulled out of the box sparkled. "Tiaras! How perfect for a princess!" Hannah thought, admiring the glittery gems. Next came magic wands, toy cars, a tic-tac-toe game, pedicure set, and chocolate candy.

Max twirled around all the stuff on the floor with his tiara propped on his head. "Please, Mommy, can't we please have some candy?" Mom smiled for the first time that day and poured some in a bowl.

Hannah fingered the pedicure set longingly until Mom noticed and told her to open it. In a minute, all three of them were giving each other pedicures and munching on chocolate candy.

Max admired his red toenails for a moment until he realized the box wasn't empty yet. "Look, Mommy! There's more!" Max shook out a pair of pajamas, slippers, craft supplies, and some pictures from Jake, Max's birthday buddy.

After studying Jake's superheroes carefully, Max went to the table and unsheathed his new markers, announcing, "I'm going to do a picture like Jake."

Mom lay back on the floor, propping her head up with her new monkey pajamas. She picked through the bowl of candy, looking for the yellow-coated chocolates.

"Mom," Hannah said, "this tiara would be perfect for a princess costume." She waited to see if Mom would pick up the hint.

Mom reached over and handed Hannah all the non-yellow candies in her hand. Then she took the tiara. Touching the twinkling rubies and diamonds Mom said, "You know, you did say you wanted to be a princess for Halloween…"

Mom had remembered! Hannah couldn't believe it, but Halloween was going to happen!

When Hannah came back to Earth, she heard Mom continuing, "…Saturday, let's go costume shopping." Shopping? Costume shopping? They never went costume shopping; they always made their costumes. This year they were going to buy their Halloween costumes?! Things were definitely looking up.

"Thank you, Rebecca!" Hannah shouted, springing up and joyfully spinning around the cluttered floor.

Mom raised her eyebrows. "Watch out for your wet polish," she warned.

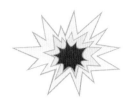

chapter 8
hair cancer

things perked up considerably around the apartment after Rebecca's box arrived. Hannah had a date for her birthday party and a costume for Halloween. Cancer wasn't going to wipe out the entire month of October after all.

One evening after Max had gone to bed, Hannah and Mom were in the living room together. Mom sat down on the sofa and pulled Hannah into her lap. Hannah knew they were about to have a really big talk. She didn't really fit in Mom's lap any more, but it was a good spot for a deep discussion.

"Cancer is pretty scary, isn't it?" Mom began.

Hannah nodded. She didn't really want to talk about cancer. The word lodged in her throat, so it was hard to talk. Even just thinking about it made her heart beat faster.

"You know, Hannah," Mom started again, "one good thing about breast cancer is that I can get rid of my breasts. Getting rid of a body part isn't anyone's first choice, but sometimes cancer is in parts of your body that the doctors can't remove. Then it's harder to treat."

"Like where?" Hannah asked curiously.

"Like in your lungs. You have to have your lungs, so if you have lung cancer, the doctors might operate to remove the tumor. But they can't take all of your lungs, which can make the treatment harder."

"Tumor?" Hannah looked puzzled.

"A tumor is what happens when the cancer cells collect together and form a mass," Mom replied. "The lump in my breast is a tumor.

"I'm going to have a bilateral mastectomy," Mom continued. "That means the doctors are going to remove both of my breasts. Another option I could choose is a lumpectomy. That's when the doctors remove just the lump and leave as much of the breast as they can. Then the woman gets radiation as an extra precaution, since not all of the breast tissue was removed."

Mom took a breath and went on, "But my lump is pretty big and my breasts are kind of small, so a lumpectomy doesn't make a lot of sense for me. There wouldn't be much breast left when they finished."

"Why both breasts? Is there cancer in the other one, too?" Hannah chewed her lip nervously.

"No," Mom shook her head and rubbed Hannah's arm reassuringly. "Having my left breast removed is called prophylactic surgery. That's a fancy word that means it's to prevent a new cancer from developing on that side.

"If you're going to have cancer, breast cancer, when it's caught early, is actually a relatively good kind to have. There's a pretty good chance the surgery alone will get rid of all of the cancer."

Hannah shook her head defiantly. "I don't think cancer is ever a good thing," she argued.

Mom smiled a little. "Yeah, but if you have to have cancer, I guess breast cancer is better than some other kinds of cancer, at least in some cases."

"What is *cancer* anyway?" Hannah asked.

"I've just learned this myself," Mom smiled at her. "Cancers are cells that don't behave like normal cells. They grow and divide and multiply abnormally, and they can travel around the body. Cancer cells can harm the body's normal cells that surround them.

"Breast cancer is a collection of deformed breast cells. Lung cancer is a collection of deformed lung cells. Once there are enough of these deformed cells, they crowd out the healthy tissue and then there aren't enough of the healthy cells to do their job properly. Or, in my case, the worry is more that the deformed cells can travel to other parts of my body, since my breasts don't really have a job to do now, like breastfeeding. Those deformed breast cells can prevent healthy cells from doing their job properly in other parts of my body."

"But how will they know if they got all of these 'deformed cells'?" Hannah asked, making air quotes with her fingers. "And," she added a little defiantly, "who is *they* anyway?"

"Well, let's start with your second question. *They* are all the doctors and lab technicians and scientists who are and will be working on me. It's pretty amazing. The doctors will do the surgery and then send the tumor to the lab to be analyzed while they are still operating on me. The lab will look at the tumor under a microscope and then send a message to the doctors who are in the operating room with me. The message will help determine if there's more surgery the doctors should do while they are already operating.

"As for getting all the deformed cells, well, that's a good question with a rather complicated answer," Mom replied. "The easy part of the answer is that I've had a bunch of tests to look for cancer in other parts of my body, and so far, none of them show anything abnormal. So that's good.

"And," Mom continued, "we won't know for a long time whether the doctors got all of the cancer cells or not. It will just depend whether or not the cancer grows anywhere else, which can take years. There's always a chance that the doctors will miss one single microscopic cell, which can then over time divide and cause problems again."

Mom looked at Hannah, who was blinking to keep tears back. "Oh, Hannah, I know. I worry about that, too." Mom blinked rapidly to stop her own tears. "But, it can happen. Cells are microscopically tiny, and on top of that, some of the deformed ones may not have fully 'deformed' yet so they may look virtually normal. No matter how thorough the doctors and lab techs are, they are human and there's no way to be one hundred percent sure they got it all…But to help keep that from happening…remember reading about the chemotherapy?"

Hannah sniffled and nodded. "That really strong medicine that will make you lose your hair and feel so sick?" she asked.

"Yep, that's the stuff," Mom agreed. "That medicine is designed to attack and kill any cancer cells that might still be in my body. That's why, even if the doctors and lab technicians think they got it all with the surgery, I'll still have chemotherapy. If any cancer cells are left, the plan is for the chemo to get them."

Mom added, "Sometimes, doctors use radiation as well. That's another type of treatment to poison and kill cancer cells. While the nurses will put chemo directly into my veins, a machine is used to send radiation through the skin to specific parts of the body. I don't think I'm going to need radiation but we won't know that for sure until after surgery."

Hannah visualized what was going on in Mom's body. "It's like a war," Hannah said with a deep breath.

"Exactly!" Mom exclaimed. "And I think I'm going to feel like I've been through a war as well."

When Hannah looked concerned, Mom reassured her, "It's just that chemo makes you really tired, in addition to making you bald."

"But, Mom," Hannah said, twisting a strand of her own hair thoughtfully, "how will the doctors know if the cancer has spread?"

Mom rubbed her forehead. "Well, after the surgery, we'll know whether my lymph system is involved."

"What's your lymph system?" Hannah looked at Mom questioningly.

Mom pointed under her arms. "One section of the lymph system is here, under my arms. The lymph system is designed to drain impurities, things that don't belong there, like cancer cells, out of your body. The problem is that as it carries these bad things out, it also gives them access to the rest of your body. On its way out of your body, a cancer cell might 'escape' and go somewhere else and set up shop."

Hannah looked confused.

41

"The lymph system acts like a highway through your body for the impurities to travel on their way out," Mom explained. "Your lymph nodes are like toll booths, stopping spots for the fluid along the lymph system. The first stop the impurities make is at the sentinel nodes. So the doctors will remove the sentinel nodes under my arms because they are the ones closest to my breast tissue, where the tumor is. The doctors will check the nodes for cancer. If the nodes don't have cancer, then most likely none of the lymph nodes have it. Then we know there's a good chance that the cancer hasn't traveled anywhere else yet."

Mom took a deep breath, "But if the lab technicians find cancer in any of the sentinel nodes, then that's the message they will send to the doctors in the operating room. The doctors will then remove as many lymph nodes in this part of my lymph system as they can find. How many lymph nodes have cancer in them helps to determine if the cancer is likely to have spread or not. It also will help the doctors decide what kind of treatment I'll need after surgery."

"So we're hoping for bankrupt cancer cells?" Hannah joked tentatively.

Now it was Mom's turn to look confused.

"Well, if the cancer is on the lymph highway, we don't want it to have enough money to get through the toll booth," Hannah explained.

Mom actually laughed. "Sort of! We would prefer the cancer never decide to take a trip on the highway, but for sure, we definitely don't want it making any premature exits!" Mom smiled. Then Mom lay her head on the back of the sofa and took a deep breath. "That's a lot of information, isn't it?"

Hannah sat quietly for a moment, picturing the war going on in Mom's body and the highway traveling underneath Mom's arm.

In a minute, Mom started talking again. "I really pray cancer is not in my lymph nodes. But," she squeezed Hannah's shoulders, "even if it is, that doesn't necessarily mean cancer has set up house somewhere else in my body."

"But, if it is in your lymph nodes?" Hannah decided she wanted to know everything.

Mom sighed. "Cancer in my lymph nodes means that the cancer is no longer just in the breast area, which is not the best news. But it still doesn't mean the cancer has spread elsewhere. It could just mean that the cancer has begun traveling on the highway but hasn't gotten off at an exit yet.

"Having cancer in more than a few lymph nodes would probably mean having more treatment than just chemotherapy. That might be a time for radiation, but I don't really know when radiation is appropriate. Some of this I'm learning just as I need to know it. It's just so much new information." Mom's eyes dropped. Hannah knew Mom was as worried as she was.

"Mom," Hannah said suddenly, "Max thinks you have cancer in your hair."

"In my hair? Why?" Mom asked startled, reaching up to pat her hair.

"Because you're going to be bald," Hannah replied.

"Oh!" Mom laughed. "So that's why he runs out of the room whenever I pick up a brush!" Mom ran her fingers through her shoulder-length hair. Hannah could remember when M.D. was a baby and Mom's hair had been short.

"I don't want to lose my hair," Mom sighed. "Not because there's cancer in my hair—there's not— but because I don't want to be bald! It's such a pain to grow hair out again, too." Mom sighed again.

"Chemo attacks any cells that grow quickly because cancer cells multiply so quickly. In this case, it's unfortunate that hair cells grow quickly, too. But the good news is that since they do grow so quickly, I'll get my hair back, or at least some of it, pretty quickly, also." Mom ruffled Hannah's light brown bob.

"Without my hair, I'm going to look pretty funny—and I'll probably be pretty tired… and," Mom sighed a little before she continued, "I'll probably throw up or at least be nauseated too. Chemo affects parts of your brain, and one of those effects is that it will probably make me feel like throwing up. The doctors will give me some medicine to help with the nausea."

When Mom took a breath, Hannah leaned back on Mom's shoulder and rubbed her hair. It felt like silk.

"I'll wear hats or maybe get a wig," Mom said.

Hannah sat straight up. "Maybe you can get my hair!" she said excitedly. "You know, the hair I donated last spring to make wigs for people with cancer? Maybe you can get a wig with my hair!"

"Wouldn't that be good luck?" Mom agreed. "At least then it would be close to the right color." Mom had dyed her hair for so long, she really didn't know what color her hair was naturally, but they had decided it was probably the same color as Hannah's.

Hannah pulled a strand of her hair next to Mom's and compared. "You'll have to get used to being darker," Hannah warned.

"I think I can do that," Mom smiled. "You know, Hannah, you can't catch cancer either. It's not contagious. Doctors don't know why some people get cancer and others don't."

"So even if you throw up, it's not like the flu?" Hannah asked.

"Nope. Even if I throw up, you can't catch cancer from me."

That was a relief. But there was one other question that had been nagging at Hannah. She tilted her head away from Mom and looked down at the floor. "Did Max or I do anything to make you get cancer?" she asked.

Mom looked at Hannah in surprise. She pulled Hannah firmly back on her lap, wrapping her tightly in her arms. "No!" Mom said emphatically. "Absolutely nothing you or your brother has ever done caused my cancer. Nothing! This isn't anyone's fault. It just happens."

Then Mom leaned into Hannah's ear and whispered," I am going to be fine."

They sat like that a long time. Hannah knew Mom didn't really know the ending of their story yet. But Hannah did know that whatever happened, their family would be fine. They had each other, and Hannah didn't need a book to tell her that.

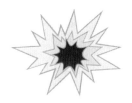

chapter 9
a camping prelude

om finally got word of when her surgery would be—the week before Halloween. This was bad news for her because she wanted the cancer out of her body as quickly as possible. But it was great news for Hannah and Max because it meant the camping trip was on!

Dad dusted off the trunk that had been in the bottom of the closet since they had moved into their apartment. Out came water bottles, a camp stove, sleeping pads, as well as a rather odd smell.

"Whew!" Mom waved at the air around her nose. "When was the last time we used that stuff?"

"Umm…I think when we climbed Mt. Mitchell—I don't know—nine years ago maybe?" Dad mused, happily digging through the rest of the crumbling pile.

"Well, in that case," Mom swooped up an armload of paraphernalia and headed to the dishwasher.

"And these!" She held the sleeping pads out at arm's length with her nose wrinkled. "Everything needs a good airing!" she said, opening them up and then propping them in front of the window.

Dad got a pad of paper and began to make a list but not before Max got in on the action.

"What's this?" Max asked, picking up one particularly noisy bundle that rattled.

"That's the cook stove," Dad said, looking up from his list.

"It doesn't look like a stove," Max said.

"Well…" Dad began putting the pieces together. Then he opened another bag and pieced together a small pot, which he put on top. "Just pretend there's a flame under it."

Max eyed the construction suspiciously. "I think I am going to get awfully hungry when we're camping," he worried. Hannah looked over. The pot was rather small.

Mom started laughing. "That, too," she said, grabbing the pot and adding it to the load in the dishwasher.

Dad wisely turned his attention to other things and dumped the tent out of its bag. "We'd better air this out too, eh?"

"How do we air it out?" Max wanted to know.

"We put it up!" Dad announced victoriously, glancing sideways to see if Mom was going to complain about having the tent take up the entire living room.

Mom was too busy at the dishwasher to notice anything else, so Dad shook the rest of the contents from the opened rucksack. A mass of leaves poured onto the carpet. Max began throwing the leaves around. Dad watched as they floated to the ground. "Souvenirs from North Carolina…" he said softly.

Then he turned his attention to the tent. "Hannah, grab that side of the canvas. That's right. Let's shake it out straight."

47

"Now, where are the tent poles?" Dad wondered, poking through all the camping equipment.

"Pow, pow, slice!" Max yelled from the dining area. He jabbed a pole at his imaginary opponent and then tried to poke the end of it through his belt loop, like a carrier.

"I'm a pirate!" Max announced, tripping over the pole, which was so long he could barely get the front end off the ground, much less through his belt loop. "Hannah, do you want to be the bad guy?"

"No. Give me that pole so we can get the tent up!"

"That's not exactly a nice way to ask," Mom commented from the kitchen.

"Please. Give. Me. That. Pole." Hannah enunciated her words very carefully so there would be no misunderstanding.

"Mommy, Hannah's still not being very nice," Max whined.

"Ah," Dad said coming through the kitchen and seeing M.D. wielding the sword. "There's one." Dad convinced Max to hand over the pole so he could watch the tent rise from the ground.

As soon as it was up, Max crawled in. "Hannah, don't you want to come in, too?"

Hannah crawled in, liking the snug, safe, cave-like feeling.

Dad busied himself on the outside. He propped the door open with the Velcro and unzipped various mesh windows to let air in. Then he stuck his head in the opening far enough to hang the gear loft, which was just a piece of mesh strung on the inside of the roof of the tent.

"Let's play camping!" Max crowed and ran off to collect his own camping gear. "Mommy, will you please get our sleeping bags?" he begged. For once Hannah thought he had a pretty good idea, so she offered to climb up on a chair to reach the bags high up in the closet.

"**W**hy?" Max whined at dinner that night. "Why can't we take the tent to Central Park and sleep in it there?"

After a pause, Max added, "To practice. To practice for our camping trip."

"We just can't," Dad said. "You just can't pitch a tent in Central Park. There might even be a law against it. I don't know."

"But Will and Hugh practiced in their tent. They got to sleep outside in their yard."

"Yeah," Hannah laughed. "But in the middle of the night, they went back to their house, remember?" She giggled thinking how silly her cousins must have looked tromping through their yard in their pjs with a flashlight."

"Anyway," Mom reminded Max, "we don't have a yard."

"But you always say Central Park is our yard, only better because it's so big," Max reminded her.

"Well," Mom stuttered a little, "yes, but…"

"Look," Dad said firmly, "we can't camp in Central Park. Period. Sorry, Buddy."

Max's lower lip trembled and his eyes narrowed. He was dangerously close to tears.

Hannah could see the sleeping bags through the open door of the tent. "Maybe," she thought out loud, "maybe we could sleep in the tent in the living room? Then if we want to get back in bed, we won't have very far to go."

Dad looked over the table at Mom. "I don't see why not," he said, thoughtfully. "But, Max-buddy, you have to go to sleep. Do you understand?"

Max nodded eagerly while Mom agreed, "Hannah, that's a great idea!"

"Mommy," Max said, his eyes wide again, "Mommy, can we please read our stories in the tent tonight, pretty please? And can we please take a flashlight, too? Will and Hugh had a flashlight!"

n obody complained about helping clean up the kitchen or getting baths after dinner that night. Max didn't want to play in the bathtub, and even Hannah took an "in-and-out" shower, not allowing herself time to relax in the hot water. Pretty soon both were snuggled in sleeping bags in between Mom and Dad with a load of bedtime stories. Dad propped a big yellow flashlight up in the gear loft so that it aimed down on them like an overhead light.

"That's what we used to do when Mom and I wanted to play cards in the tent at night," Dad explained, obviously very satisfied with the situation.

Hannah moved her fingers through the light, making shadows dance on the sleeping bags. "Look, a bunny!" she said wiggling two fingers.

Dad moved his thumb and index finger to make a dog bark.

Max started rolling around in his sleeping bag, banging into Hannah. "Ow! He hit me! Mom! Make him stop!" Hannah glared at her brother. "If you don't stop, I'm not going to sleep in here," Hannah threatened, knowing M.D. would be too scared to sleep in the tent alone.

"Even if you sleep in your bed, Mom and Dad will be right here," Max said smugly.

"Oh, no, I only sleep in a sleeping bag when I'm actually outdoors," Mom corrected him. "Not when my nice comfortable bed is mere feet away..." She nodded down the hallway toward her and Dad's bedroom. Quickly, before Max could protest any further, Mom added, "Story time," and cracked open one of Max's books.

In the middle of one of the stories, Max shifted his gaze from the pictures to Mom's chest. "Mommy," he said, snuggling up to her, "how will they get rid of your canker?"

"...ssser, cancer," Hannah hissed.

"They'll cut it out," Mom told him.

"All of it?" Max wanted to know.

"We hope all of it. Then I'll have that strong medicine..."

"Oh that stuff that will make you be bald. The kem, kemo, kemo-sabi?" Max looked to Hannah for help.

"Chemotherapy," Hannah told him authoritatively.

"The chemotherapy," Mom agreed. "will hopefully kill any of the cancer they might accidentally miss when they cut it out."

"Will they put your chest back on?" Max looked worried.

"Sort of," Mom said. "They'll do something called reconstruction."

"What's that?" Hannah asked interestedly. No one had mentioned anything about reconstruction.

"Well, first they'll put something kind of like water balloons under the skin of my chest. The nurses will put a little water in the balloons each time I see the doctor. The water will make the balloons expand or get bigger. That will stretch my skin and muscle nice and slowly. When they are all blown up and my skin has a chance to get used to being stretched, I'll have another surgery. The balloons will come out, and they'll put in implants. They will be my new chest. It will look a lot like my old chest," Mom finished up.

She glanced over at Dad with a funny smile on her face. "Did you ever think we'd be talking to our kids about implants?"

"Will it hurt?" Max wanted to know.

"Yes," Dad said. "it won't hurt forever, but it will definitely hurt for a while. We'll have to take special care of Mom right after her surgery." He reached over Hannah and Max and rubbed Mom's shoulder.

"How will it be different from your old chest?" Max asked.

"Well," Mom thought a minute. "My chest right now is made up of cells that are alive. The implants won't be alive, so cancer can't grow in them. They are made of a material called silicone—it feels kind of like gummy bears and when it breaks, it looks like a gummy bear, a little gooey in the middle."

"Does it taste good?" Max wanted to know.

"I don't think so," Mom laughed.

"What else?" Max persisted.

"Well....I won't have much feeling where my breasts are now. That will be kind of weird."

"You mean if I hit you here," Max said pointing to Mom's chest, "you won't feel it?"

"I will be very mad if you hit Mom there or anywhere!" Dad broke in.

"You're not supposed to hit, M.D.," Hannah reminded him.

"But if Mommy won't feel it, why can't I hit her?" Max protested.

"You don't hit Mom or anyone," Dad said. "Is that clear?"

Max nodded soberly.

Mom added, "I won't have much feeling right where my breasts are, but I think the rest of my chest will be pretty sore."

"And it'll probably hurt under your arms where they have to take out your lymph nodes," Hannah added, thinking about their conversation the other night.

Mom nodded. "Yeah, I think mostly it's all going to take some getting used to." After a minute she said, "So should we say our prayers?"

They sat quietly a minute after they prayed together. Hannah asked God privately, "Please let Mom get better, and please, God, keep the cancer out of her lymph nodes."

Max added aloud, "Please, God, don't let the canker hurt my mommy."

53

When Hannah squinted up at Mom, she thought she saw a tear on her cheek. Dad must have seen it too, because he reached over them and rubbed Mom's hair.

"hannah, Hannah," M.D. whispered through the dark, his plea bouncing off the canvas ceiling. "Hanny…"

"What?! I'm trying to sleep!"

Max found the flashlight in the gear loft and flicked it on.

"Hannah, do you think the doctor will save the water balloons from Mommy's chest so we can take them to the park? There's going to be two of them so we won't even have to share."

"Max, turn off the flashlight and go to sleep!"

He turned off the flashlight and dropped it back in the gear loft.

"Hannah?"

"What? Enough already! I want to go to sleep!"

"Hannah, I'm scared. I want to get in my bed. Please?" Max felt for Hannah's hand.

"Get the flashlight and let's go," Hannah said, pretending to be stern but secretly a little relieved. The wooden floor under the sleeping bag and mat was pretty hard, and her back was beginning to ache.

Mom was snoring as they crept down the hall. When they got to their room, Hannah tucked the covers around M.D. and crawled up the ladder.

"Max," Hannah leaned over from the top bunk. "Max, I love you." But he was already asleep.

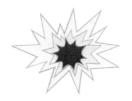

chapter 10
dessert swap

the week before the camping trip dragged on forever. Ms. Calde put the history project at the top of her priority list, and Hannah's class had group meetings every day.

Hannah couldn't decide which site to pick for her individual report. She was torn between Trinity Church and Thomas Paine Park. There was definitely more information available about Trinity Church, but she thought the challenge just might make the park more interesting.

Hannah decided she really needed to see the sites in person before she could pick one to research. Mom had agreed to take her downtown, but they couldn't find an afternoon to go. Between soccer practice, piano, and pre-op tests for Mom, only Friday was left. Hannah didn't want to go on Friday because she didn't want to run late in case Dad could get out of work a little early to leave for the camping trip. She and Mom blocked out the following Monday on the calendar posted on the refrigerator, with the caveat they would go later if something else came up. Until then, Hannah felt at loose ends about her part of the project.

Lydia's growing possessiveness also stretched out that eternal week. Hannah was beginning to wonder why she had wanted Lydia to be her best friend so badly. Sure, Lydia was pretty with her super-long, almost white hair, huge blue eyes, and wide smile. She carried herself impressively tall and straight, too. Just thinking about her made Hannah throw her shoulders back.

Lydia had also impressed everyone in the class the first day of school with her loud proclamation that she was reading "T" level books. When Hannah really thought about it, though, she realized she had felt like being chosen to be Lydia's best friend was a badge of honor.

Now, however, Hannah was tired of being with just Lydia all the time. She had tried to sit between Mary and Lydia at lunch so she could talk to both of them, but that hadn't gone so well.

Scottie had been sitting across the table from them when he reached over and snatched one of Mary's chocolate chip oatmeal cookies.

"Hey! My grandma made those!" Mary exclaimed.

Mary eyed Scottie frantically as he turned the cookie on its side and rolled it down the table. Just as it was careening towards the edge, he put his arm around Josh's back and dramatically scooped the cookie up in mid-air.

Hannah laughed and reassured Mary, " Don't worry. He won't eat it. Scottie's just a clown." Then she whispered conspiratorially in Mary's ear, "And a bit of a show-off."

Scottie knelt up on the lunch bench and bowed low over the table, offering the cookie back to Mary on the palm of his hand. Mary smiled shyly and broke the cookie in half. She offered one of the pieces to Scottie.

Just then, Lydia teased, "You should try this instead." She dangled a large, fragrant cookie in front of Scottie's nose. "It's pumpkin chocolate chip. I made them last night. They're really good." Glancing at Mary, Lydia added, "I've got two, so you can have that whole one if you want."

Mary turned red and looked down at the one and a half cookies still in her lunch box.

Scottie took both Mary and Lydia's offerings. "Thanks! Hey, Hannah, what do you have for dessert?"

Hannah dug around in her lunch box. "Ummm… let's see… I have five Hershey kisses!" she finally announced, holding the chocolates up triumphantly.

Scottie leaned down the table, "Anybody who wants to, put your dessert in the middle and we'll split it up. That way everyone will get a variety." He spread out a napkin.

Several other kids added contributions to the napkin, and Scottie dropped the cookies on it as well. "OK, Hannah," Scottie said, "you do the dividing. You're the most fair."

Everybody nodded and, except for Lydia, grinned when Hannah passed around the napkin heaped with individual helpings from their dessert smorgasbord.

Licking the last morsel off his lips just as the recess whistle blew, Scottie announced on the way to the trash cans, "Same thing tomorrow—dessert swap if you want!"

Hannah and Lydia got outside before Mary. Lydia flipped her thick hair over her shoulders and then sniffed, "I meant for Scottie to have my whole cookie, not just a mere smidgen."

In the bright sun, Hannah squinted at Lydia, whose hair was sparkling in the light. Hannah felt her own short bob. Why had she agreed to cut her hair again last month? Now it would be forever before it was long enough for a ponytail.

Lydia spotted Mary running in their direction and wrinkled her nose. "She's going to want to play something," Lydia said, jerking her thumb in Mary's direction.

Hannah peered at Lydia again. She knew Lydia didn't like playing games any more. She preferred to talk, usually about someone, or organize a new club, of which she was always the president.

Mary nodded at Lydia as she reached them. "Your cookies were really good. You're lucky your mom cooks with you. I don't remember the last time my mom turned on an oven. If I asked her to teach me how to cook, she'd just send me down the street to the bakery!"

"My mom didn't teach me to cook," Lydia replied coolly. " I learned from a cookbook."

"Wow!" Hannah said. "Do you get to use knives and handle hot stuff from the oven too?"

"Yeah," Lydia rolled her eyes, considering this a boring discussion. "Sure. My mom doesn't even know I cook. I do it when she's not home."

"I'm allowed to use a paring knife but not the bigger ones. And I'm not allowed to turn on the oven if Mom's not there," Hannah began. Then she started suddenly, "But she's never not there. I mean," Hannah fumbled, flustered, "there's always a grown-up around, even if Mom isn't there."

Mary nodded in agreement, but Lydia shook her head. "I can't believe your mom won't leave you alone. She must not trust you."

Hannah was silent. Lydia was the first kid she knew who stayed alone. A few, like Carl, had older siblings who sometimes babysat for them, but no one stayed alone. Was it because Mom didn't trust her?

Scottie caught Hannah staring off in the distance and waved her over to their game of *Steal the Bacon*. Lydia saw him, too. "You go," Lydia prompted Mary, pointing to Scottie. "Hannah and I are busy here."

Mary shot Hannah a puzzled glance, and Hannah looked at the ground, feeling very uncomfortable. When Hannah didn't say anything, Mary shrugged and sprinted over to the game in progress.

Hannah squirmed. Lydia had been pretty mean and Hannah knew she should say something. But she didn't want to cross Lydia and unleash her wrath. Besides, Lydia often found interesting projects on the Internet at night, and Hannah really wanted to see what she had printed off last night.

The page Lydia handed her had fake fingernails printed on it. "Color them and we'll cut them out and tape them over our real nails," Lydia said.

Hannah looked down at her own fingernails, which Mom made her keep short and bare. Lydia always had beautifully shaped and painted nails. Lydia noticed Hannah's hands, too. "Then you can pretend you have pretty nails."

They sat down on a bench, and Lydia pulled out an assortment of markers for them to work with. "Now be daring," Lydia said, beginning to stripe her own set.

"**m**om, can you get me up a little early tomorrow morning?" Hannah asked before bed.

"Sure, but why?" Mom asked as she looked up at Hannah in surprise from the game of *Uno* she and Max were playing. "You hate getting up early!"

"Oh, I just need to do something," Hannah replied vaguely. Then she slipped into their room to work on her fingernails.

"**W**hy can't I wear these to school?" Hannah demanded the next morning at breakfast, waving her red-striped fingertips around wildly.

"Because…," Mom stuttered, glancing in Dad's direction for support.

Hannah could tell Dad was trying to hide a smile, which made her even madder.

"How are you going to hold a pencil, much less write, with those things stuck on your hand?" Mom argued.

"Like this!" Hannah flew up from the table, grabbed a pen from the kitchen counter, and demonstrated. The paper on her index finger bent back slightly, but she thought it still looked realistic enough.

Mom softened a little. "Hannah, if you want, we'll paint your nails tonight, but you can't wear paper taped to your fingers to school."

"But I need to wear them today!" Now Hannah was getting desperate. Lydia would have her nails on this morning, Hannah was sure. "Besides, even if we do paint them tonight, we can't make them fancy or do stripes!"

"True," Mom agreed. "But…"

Dad intervened calmly. "Liz, tell me what you think, but I really don't see why Hannah can't wear them to school today."

Hannah's shoulders slumped in relief.

Dad shifted his gaze from Mom to Hannah. "Just today," he added firmly, "and if there's a problem doing school work, the nails go away."

Hannah nodded vigorously.

After a pause, Mom said shortly, "OK, but any problems writing and those things get trashed!"

"OK," Hannah agreed.

a fter lunch, Hannah noted happily that Mom hadn't skimped on the Hershey kisses today, so there were plenty to share. She reached, quite elegantly she thought, for her dessert portion with her newly manicured hand.

"Why do you have paper taped to your fingers?" Scottie asked curiously.

Lydia, who had just arrived at school from an orthodontist's appointment, giggled and reached for her portion, too. Her fingers were also freshly manicured, but under the cafeteria's fluorescent lights, they gleamed with real red polish

Hannah's face flamed in the face of Lydia's treachery.

Glancing down at her own hands now, Hannah saw bits of scotch tape anchoring rough-edged paper pieces to plain-Jane fingers. The stripes weren't quite straight and in a couple of places, color strayed outside the lines. "Like a three-year-old," Hannah thought angrily, pulling off the nails and crumpling them into a ball under the table.

Mary was already playing when Hannah got outside for recess. Hannah sat down on a bench with a thud.

"Why'd you take off your nails?" Lydia suddenly materialized beside Hannah.

"Because they looked stupid," Hannah muttered.

"No, they didn't," Lydia said, making sure to wave her perfectly done hand under Hannah's nose.

"Yes," Hannah gritted her teeth, "they did." Why, she wondered, had she argued with Mom about something so dumb?

"Whatever," Lydia said tossing her trademark mane over her shoulder and walking over to where Mary and Scottie were playing *Steal the Bacon* with the others.

Hannah got only a little bit of satisfaction when she noticed how awkward and stiff Lydia looked standing on the periphery of the game already in progress. It wasn't as much comfort as she would have liked it to be.

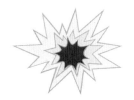

chapter 11
camping

"**d**addy, why isn't Mommy coming with us?" Max asked as he twisted around in his booster seat to wave to Mom on the sidewalk one more time.

"Max," Hannah replied impatiently, "you know why!"

"She said she wanted some peace and quiet. Daddy, what's 'peace and quiet'?"

"Getting away from you," Hannah muttered, looking out the window.

"Peace and quiet is just what it sounds like," Dad said from the driver's seat. "Quiet—no noise, and peace—nice and restful. Mom has had a lot going on recently and with her surgery coming up, she just needed some time on her own. But think of all the stuff you'll have to tell her when we get back Sunday night!"

"What kind of stuff?"

"What kind of stuff?!" Dad exclaimed. "What kind of stuff? Just you wait!"

"Roasting marshmallows, sleeping in a sleeping bag, seeing Will, Hugh, and Jimmy, fishing," Hannah ticked off the adventures awaiting them on her fingers.

"Oh, right," Max said, "And staying up late and making pancakes on the cook stove and putting up the tent and..." M.D. floundered trying to think of more things.

"Seeing stars, going hiking, not having to take a bath, sleeping in our clothes, seeing all of your cousins from both sides of the family..." Dad added from the front seat.

"You know," Hannah reminded Max, "Jenny and Liam, Will, Hugh, and Jimmy, and..."

"No bath?" Max interrupted her grinning. "Sleeping in our clothes? That's silly! We prob'ly couldn't do that if Mommy came."

"Seeing stars," Hannah mused, watching the lights of the city fall behind them. They didn't see too many stars at home because of all the city lights. "I looked at my calendar. We're supposed to get a full moon tomorrow," she remarked.

"A full moon? Really?" Dad said. "That's a good omen."

"Who are the *Oh Mens*? Are they coming, too?" Max piped up.

"*Mens*? What *mens*? What are you talking about?" Hannah asked. Max never got things straight.

"The *oh mens* Daddy was talking about."

"Omen, Silly! Not *oh mens*. An omen is like..." Hannah couldn't think of a good synonym.

"Sign," Dad supplied. "A full moon is a good sign— we'll probably have good weather."

As they crossed the bridge into New Jersey, Max waved through the window. "Bye, bye New York City! Camping here we come!"

the next morning Hannah woke up before M.D., which was really weird. Chilly, she slithered out of her sleeping bag. She grabbed a fleece and kept sliding towards the door. There sure wasn't much room in the tent with the sleeping bags out and stuff scattered everywhere.

When Dad heard Hannah fumbling with the zipper, he helped her escape through the doorway. Squinting in the bright sunshine, Hannah saw lots of people, kids and grownups, sitting on the rocks around the campfire.

Jenny rushed over and swooped her up into a big hug. "Hannah! You've gotten taller just since August." Hannah grinned. All of her pants were getting too short.

Jenny carried Hannah, still enveloped in a bear hug, over to the fire. "Hot chocolate?" When Hannah nodded, Jenny dumped hot cocoa mix from a packet into a mug and poured steaming hot water over it. Then she pulled out a second packet. "Marshmallows!" Jenny announced in a very satisfied tone.

After she pointed to a rock for Hannah to sit on, Jenny pulled out another packet from a grocery bag with a wink and said, "When you eat those up, here are some more." Jenny was the kind of person who understood the importance of marshmallows.

Next, Jenny pointed to a skinny boy and a curly-headed girl also sitting on the rocks. "This is my nephew, Fatty, and his sister, Sally, who's..." here Jenny gently elbowed the girl and smiled broadly, "...also my niece." Hannah thought that Fatty had a really funny name, given how skinny he was.

After a minute, Jenny added, gesturing at the other kids slurping hot chocolate on the rocks, "And these are their friends, Rob, Jason, and Carmen." All the kids kind of nodded at each other, not knowing what to say.

But everyone definitely knew how to answer Jenny's next question, "Who else needs more marshmallows?"

Suddenly, the doorway of the biggest tent in the campground flung open, and the Bennett cousins poured out. "You already know who we are!" they shouted, dancing around the fire. "Yum! Hot chocolate and marshmallows!" It was the first time the Bennett cousins from both sides of the family had met. Marshmallows cemented the tentative familial relationship.

By the time M.D. emerged from the tent, everyone had gone canoeing except for the Bennetts. Dad glanced at his watch, "Wow! I'm going to tell Mom we need to put a sleeping bag on your bed at home. You've never slept this late! Now what should we do today?"

"Where's your mom?" Will asked at the campfire that night.

"She stayed home because of the canker," Max told him.

"*Cancer*, not canker," Hannah hissed at him, thinking Max would never get that word right. Then Hannah corrected him, "She didn't stay home because of the cancer…"

"Oh, right," Max interrupted her, "she stayed home because I am too loud and she wanted to sleep."

"Peace and quiet," Hannah explained to Will. "She wanted some peace and quiet."

Will nodded. "Yeah, sometimes my mom needs that, too."

"Mommy's gonna be bald," Max told Will.

Will raised his eyebrows at this announcement.

"Because of the canker." Max added.

"*Cancer*," Hannah said again. Then she added, "But just for a little while. Her hair'll grow back."

Suddenly they heard an excited yelp, and a circle of light started swirling around in the big tent. "Look guys!" Hugh hollered from inside. "It's a light show!"

Will jumped up. "Grab your flashlights! Party in the tent!" he yelled.

Shadows around the fire bobbed furiously while all the kids collected their flashlights and ran into the big tent. They danced around, jumping over sleeping bags, bumping into each other, and bouncing off the ceiling of the tent until Jimmy, the youngest Bennett cousin, fell over and got stepped on. Aunt Kath made everyone settle down while she fished Jimmy out from the pile of kids and gear.

Then Fatty started telling jokes. Hannah still couldn't believe people called him Fatty and he didn't mind. She shook her head. He wasn't anywhere near fat!

"Knock, knock."

"Who's there?"

"Orange."

"Orange who?"

"Orange you glad you didn't get stepped on?"

Groans all around, and then Will asked, "Why is the library so tall?"

"I already know that one!" Rob answered. "Because it has so many stories!"

"OK, OK. So, how do you make a hot dog stand?"

"Take away its chair!" Will pumped his arm in the air.

Somebody else yelled, "Why do porcupines never lose games?"

"Because they always have the most points!"

Then Max chimed in, "Hey, you guys listen to me—why did the chicken cross the road?"

Hannah rolled her eyes. Half the time M.D.'s jokes didn't make any sense. And the ones that did make sense had been out on the joke circuit for a long time.

"To get to the other side. That's an old one." The older boys brushed Max off.

"No, that's not why. It's because he wanted pizza!" Max cracked himself up. He was right—no one guessed his answer.

Instead, everyone groaned again. "That doesn't make any sense!"

Will said, "Hugh does that, too—tells jokes that don't make sense."

Max's eyes got very tiny, and Hannah knew he was about to cry. Just then Hugh shined his flashlight up from underneath a sleeping bag, making ghosts dance on the walls of their temporary home. The wind rattled above the tent fly.

Fatty disguised his voice in a creepy whine. "There was an old, broken down house on a deserted hill, many miles from the nearest town. No one lived there, except for one lonesome—GHOST!" At that, Fatty gave an eerie shriek. Heads bumped as kids jumped in terror.

"The ghost liked to hide under things." Someone moved a flashlight in slow, spooky circles.

"If you were lucky, you knew where he was because you could see just a bit of his white ghostly-ness. But if you were unlucky, all was black…" Fatty's voice trailed off and the flashlight clicked in the silence, leaving only darkness.

In a moment, Fatty picked up the story again, "And you didn't know where he was!"

"Whoooooo…" a voice hollowed through the air.

Max whimpered. "I want my mommy."

Hannah moved closer to him and put her arm across his back. "It's OK, Buddy. It's just a story."

Max burrowed into Hannah, and she could feel his head shaking. She knew that under the sleeping bag, his eyes were filling up. "I want Mommy!"

"Mom's at home, but Dad's right by the fire. You can go to him."

Fatty whistled his hollow, ghostly sound again.

Max trembled harder. "I want you to go with me," he sniffed, grabbing tightly at Hannah's hand. She knew Max was really scared and that she should help him out of the tent. She wasn't all that unhappy to leave the darkness herself. It was getting kind of creepy in there.

Hannah and Max stumbled over the assortment of kids and through the doorway. As they left the haunted tent, Hannah could see a billion stars. "Wow!" she breathed.

Max looked up too. He pointed to the moon. "Hannah! Look! It's a full moon!"

"Wow!" she breathed again. The sky in the city sure didn't look anything like this.

the sky in the city wasn't black, and it didn't glitter with faraway diamonds, but the Bennetts were pretty happy to see the neon lights that announced they were almost home the next night. They couldn't wait to tell Mom about fishing, marshmallows, and the party in the tent. M.D. couldn't wait to tell her that they'd slept in their clothes and that they hadn't had a bath.

"I love camping," Max said as Dad turned the corner on to our street. "But my favorite place in the whole wide world is East 77th Street!"

Suddenly, his voice started trembling. "Daddy, I don't want to go to Heaven."

"Why not, Buddy?"

"Because if you go to Heaven, you don't get to come to East 77th Street."

When Hannah glanced at Max, his eyes were tiny, little slivers. She could tell the tears were lined up and ready to spill.

Dad said, "But, Max, Heaven is even better than East 77th Street! Can you imagine that? Even better. Once you get to Heaven, you won't want to come back to East 77th Street!"

"I don't want to go away from East 77th Street," Max sniffled. Then he said, "Is East 77th Street Mommy's favorite place in the whole wide world? Or does she want to go to Heaven?"

Hannah could feel Dad thinking hard. "Well," Dad said, "she wants to go to Heaven some day. But right now, she wants to live on East 77th Street with you and Hannah and me.

"It's OK not to be ready to go to Heaven yet," Dad added. "Earth is a pretty cool place to be, and we should enjoy it while we're here. But someday, when it's time, we'll go to

Heaven, and it will be so amazing, so much fun, we can't even picture it.

"Anyway, none of us is going to Heaven right now. Right now we're going home to East 77th Street and tell Mom all about camping! We have to get her all excited so she will want to go with us the next time."

Max's eyes opened wide and he said, "Yeah, just as soon as she gets rid of her cank...ser!"

"Closer, Buddy," Dad laughed.

Hannah couldn't help muttering, "Cancer." Maybe Max did need to say it one hundred times. Or even more. Just not with her around.

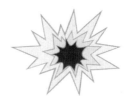

chapter 12
long-distance hugs

he buzz of the alarm Wednesday morning reminded Hannah that something was going on. As she burrowed deeper under the comforter and yelled for Max to turn off the clock, Hannah was almost relieved that the day had finally arrived but she wasn't sure why.

Max climbed up the bunk bed ladder and poked at her feet with a toy golf club. "Stop it!" Hannah shrieked, throwing the covers back just far enough to glower at him. He stepped back and promptly fell off the ladder, landing hard on the floor. When she peeked over the railing to check on him, Hannah saw the rumpled sheets on the extra bed in their room. She could hear water running in the bathroom. Oh yeah, Papa was visiting—he must be getting ready.

Suddenly, Max yelped, "Look, Hannah! We've got new shirts!"

Hannah peered over the bed railing and saw Max sitting on top of two new shirts, one of which seemed to be lighting up. They had a note nestled between them.

As Hannah came down from her bed, Max picked up the note, announcing, "I'm going to read it! I know I can—this right here says 'I love you!' Look, there's the I, and here's the love part, and," he jabbed his finger at the paper, "that's the you. I love you! I can read! Hannah, I can really read!"

Max spun around the floor, tripped on a stray toy, and fell over on to his shirt, which immediately lit up again. Hannah rolled her eyes. She was sure more tears were in the making. Instead, Max gasped, "Hannah! My shirt lights up! Oh, wow!" He punched at the picture on his shirt a few more times. "I'm wearing this today! Does yours do anything?"

Before Hannah could answer, Papa came in the room and picked up the note Max had dropped in his excitement.

"Dear Hannah and Max," Papa read. "Wear your new shirts today and you'll feel me giving you a big hug all day. I love you! Love, Mom." Oh. Hannah's heart sank. Surgery. Today was the day of surgery. Mom wasn't here. She and Dad were at the hospital.

"Hannah, put your shirt on!" Max insisted. "Put it on! Does it do anything?" Hannah picked up the shirt Mom had chosen for her and fingered the neckline gently. It was pink, her favorite color, and it had tiny beads and sequins sewn in a circle around the top. Hannah loved sparkles.

Then Hannah felt her own tears well up. She was embarrassed for Papa to see them, but now with her new shirt, she knew she was going to think about Mom all day. She wouldn't even be able to pretend that everything was normal. She had to be prepared for an awful day.

73

"I like your shirt," Mary said shyly to Hannah on the way upstairs to the classroom.

"Thanks," Hannah replied shortly, looking for Lydia over Mary's shoulder.

When she saw Mary's eyes fall, Hannah added softly, "It's new. My mom gave it to me."

Mary smiled. "The sparkles are really pretty."

Just then Lydia breezed up to them. "Hi, Hannah. Do you like my new hair clip?"

Mary looked down again.

"Hi Lydia," Hannah said, suddenly feeling uncomfortable as Mary walked to her seat. "Yeah, it's very, ah, very big."

Lydia swished her ponytail dramatically as she made her entrance into the classroom. Everybody watched. Everybody always watched Lydia. Lydia never just walked. Lydia always made an entrance.

Ms. Calde called for History Group Meetings. Hannah flushed. She hadn't done anything on her part of the project yet. She busied herself pulling supplies out of her desk.

Scottie turned to her, "Come on, Hannah." He reached over to drag her desk into the group he, Mary, and Sam were already forming. "Hey! I can do it!" Hannah snapped.

Scottie raised his eyebrows in surprise. He shrugged and turned back to their cluster as Hannah rotated her desk around. When she sat down, one of the sequins on her shirt winked in the light. Scottie held up his hand, pretending to be blinded by the glare, and the others laughed.

Hannah dropped her head and shrank down in her desk. What were the doctors doing to Mom now? She crossed her arms in front of her and squeezed. There, that was a hug from

Mom. That should make her feel better. But instead, she found herself blinking back more tears.

Sam started their meeting by saying he thought they really needed to make an outline of the important events, that way each of their parts could highlight a piece of the outline. Sam, Hannah was learning, was very organized.

Scottie grabbed his pencil. "So what were the big events during the Revolutionary War?" he asked.

As Sam bent his head over his notes, Mary touched Hannah's arm. "Are you OK?" she asked, concerned.

Hannah shrugged and nodded, unable to look up.

After a moment, Mary asked, "Have you already picked your place to research?"

Hannah shook her head, still looking down. "I haven't been able to get downtown yet."

Just then Scottie broke in, "What do you guys think?"

"About what?" Mary wanted to know as she and Hannah looked up.

"These," Scottie waved his hand over some sentences he and Sam were working on, "are what we think are the really important events. We think it should start with Thomas Paine. That's you, right, Hannah?"

Hannah nodded mutely. Scottie waited a minute, expecting her to say something. When she didn't, he resumed, "But how much of all the stuff going on in Massachusetts should we include? It's not part of the Revolution in New York City."

Out of the corner of her eye, Hannah watched Lydia's white-blonde ponytail with its huge glittering bow swish in rhythm with her mouth. Lydia always had something to say.

Mary brought Hannah back to their group's work, "Well, we have to tell some of what was going on in Massachusetts so everyone will know why New York was involved at all."

"Yeah," Sam agreed. "That's part of the research we all do."

All four of them nodded in agreement.

"Then, Hannah, do you want to do something on Thomas Paine and Thomas Paine Park to kind of get us going in New York?" Sam suggested.

Hannah nodded at Sam. "Sure, I can do that." Then there was silence.

The four of them looked at each other awkwardly, waiting for someone to say something. When nothing was forthcoming, Scottie shot Hannah a questioning look, and then said, "So what event should we put next?"

By the time the meeting time was over, the Revolutionary War Group had a list of important events and each of the members had a specific research project. They also had the distinct feeling that something was not right.

"Are you OK?" Scottie scooted his head under Hannah's elbow as they were turning their desks back towards the front. He twisted around and rested the back of his head on the surface of her desk. With his eyebrows raised in a question mark, he looked up at her from his position lying across her desk.

Hannah nodded.

"Are you sure?" There was another long pause. "You didn't have much to say back there," Scottie added as he righted himself and moved back to his own desk.

"I haven't done anything for the project yet," Hannah said through her teeth. "But, don't worry, I will."

"You don't have to do Thomas Paine if you don't want."

"I'll do Thomas Paine!" Hannah snapped.

Scottie shrugged. "Whatever," he said, nonchalantly.

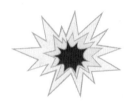

chapter 13
the hospital

On Friday morning, Dad asked if Hannah and Max wanted to go see Mom at the hospital after school. Max thought this was a great idea, but Hannah was nervous.

Hospitals were serious places. She worried about how sick Mom was going to look. She worried about how sore Mom was going to be—if she hugged Mom, would it hurt Mom? She worried she might touch something important and break it. Then the doctors would be mad, at her and maybe at Mom too.

She was also worried about seeing Mom bald. Even if hair was just hair and not really that important, Mom was still going to look pretty strange.

Hannah decided she really didn't want to go after all, but Dad wouldn't take no for an answer. He said Mom would be really disappointed if they didn't come. But he did promise they didn't have to stay very long.

As Hannah expected, the hospital was a big, scary place. There were a lot of really old, sick-looking people in wheel-chairs with all sorts of tubes and wires attached to them. The scariest ones didn't have hair. Their shiny, smooth heads made them look like aliens. No eyebrows either. Nothing was there, it seemed, to make them look human. Hannah prayed Mom would still look human.

The closer they got to Mom's room, the slower Hannah went. Finally Dad turned and took her hand. "Hannah, what's up? Come on. You'll see. It's not that bad."

Max bounded into Mom's room. "Mommy!" Hannah and Dad heard him shriek as they followed him down the hall. "Mommy! You have hair!"

Hannah peeked in from the doorway. Mom looked like a pile of spaghetti, all arms and legs and tubes, as she moved in slow motion from the bed to hug Max.

Afterwards, Mom reached up to touch her hair. "Why wouldn't I have hair?" she asked, puzzled.

"You're supposed to be bald!" Max looked a little disappointed. "You know, from the cankser…"

"Oh. I see," Mom nodded. "I'll be bald when I start the chemotherapy. But that's not for a few weeks. I get to keep my hair for a little while yet. It needs a good washing, but at least it's my hair."

"First, Mom has to get well from the surgery," Dad interjected.

Mom stood up slowly, rolling a pole behind her. But she definitely still had hair and eyebrows and even eyelashes. No matter how strange everything else looked, Mom still had hair. That was a relief.

"Hannah! I've missed you! How was school?" The tube, attached to both her arm and the bag on the pole, snaked around Hannah as Mom gingerly gave her a hug.

Hannah tried to be so very careful. Mom looked so fragile and she moved so delicately that Hannah was really afraid she'd hurt her. Mom smiled at Hannah as she rubbed Hannah's back gently. "I may look like I'll break, but I won't. I promise."

Then Mom patted the bed. "You guys jump up here. There's a big room upstairs with crafts for the patients, and I got some stuff for you to do." Mom pushed the rolling table in front of Max and Hannah and gave them glue and little tiles and a piece of cardboard to make a design.

Then Mom sank into the chair beside the bed. Suddenly she looked pretty tired. Dad adjusted her IV pole to the side of the chair while she asked all kinds of questions about school and how the rest of the week had gone.

Max finished his pattern and started looking around for something else to do. Mom told him to lie down on the bed. "But, Mommy, I don't want to take a nap! I'm too old for naps now," he protested.

"No nap," Mom promised. "Just try it." So Max stretched out behind Hannah, who was perched on the edge of the bed. Then he turned his eyes suspiciously to Mom. She started pushing buttons on a remote from her chair.

"Oh…" Max giggled as the whole bed went up and down, and then both the head of the bed and the foot of the bed moved up and down separately.

Hannah hopped off the bed to watch him.

"Can I do it? Please?" Max begged.

Mom handed over the controls, and M.D. immediately folded himself into the bed by raising both the head and the foot at the same time. Then he squished himself together, his nose touched his knees, and his feet poked out over the top of the mattress. Max offered Hannah the remote. "You wanna turn?"

She didn't, actually. Now she was sitting on the edge of Mom's chair, more than a little scared the bed might get stuck that way. Then how would Mom sleep? Mom looked like she really needed some sleep.

Everybody, including the nurse who had come in to take Mom's blood pressure, was laughing at Max. Finally Dad said, "Hannah can't very well take a turn with you sandwiched in there like that. Flatten yourself out, Buddy."

After a lot of experimental button-pushing, Max finally got the bed back to its original position and offered Hannah the remote one more time. She shook her head stiffly, afraid to move too much on the chair and bump Mom. What she really wanted was to get out of the hospital altogether.

After a minute, Mom said, "Well, if you really don't want to try it, Hannah, I might climb in."

Dad helped Mom shift from the chair back into the bed and covered her up with the blanket. "That's better," Mom smiled. "Where's that remote? I need to raise my head."

"I'll do it, Mommy!" Max announced as he started to mash a button with his finger.

Dad stopped him. "No, Buddy. Mom needs to do it herself. If you go too fast, it might hurt her."

"I'll go slow, Daddy. I promise."

"Max, give the remote to Mom." Dad ordered in a no-funny-business-allowed tone.

Max reluctantly relinquished the controls, and Mom raised the head of the bed.

81

Now that Mom was lying in the bed, Hannah could see the bandages wrapped around Mom's chest. She also had more tubes attached to bulbs that dangled inside her hospital gown. When Mom saw Hannah looking at them, she said, "Those are my drains. The fluid that normally goes into the lymph nodes has to drain here until it figures out new channels to travel. And also some blood," Mom added. "That's what makes it red."

"Will you have the drains forever?" Max wanted to know.

"Oh, my gosh, no!" Mom exclaimed. "That would be miserable! No. Just until they stop collecting fluid. Maybe only a week or so," she said hopefully.

The drains reminded Hannah of the lymph nodes. "Mom?" she asked tentatively. Hannah shored up her remaining courage. "Mom, did you have cancer in your lymph nodes?"

Mom dropped her eyes for a second and then raised her head to look Hannah in the eye. "In one node, Hannah. Unfortunately, I had it in one node. But they took out all the other nodes that they could find, and they were all clean. That's the good news."

She smiled at Hannah and motioned for her to come closer. "The doctor came by this morning, and they really think they got all the cancer in the surgery. Once I feel a bit better from the surgery, I'll start the chemotherapy, just to make sure. Then, maybe, things will start getting back to normal. That would be good, eh?"

"What's normal?" Max asked, as he started pushing the buttons on the IV pole.

"Not you, that's for sure," Hannah thought, as Dad grabbed Max's hand away from the IV pole. Normal seemed awfully far away.

"Uh, normal is when we go home so Mom can get some rest and you can't do any damage here!" Dad said, ushering Hannah and Max towards the door.

"Hey, wait a minute!" Mom said. "I need goodbye hugs!"

Max flew into her arms. Hannah was pretty sure she saw Mom wince when Max put his forehead to her chest.

"Hey, Hannah-Banana! Come here! Give me a proper hug." Hannah came over and stood stiffly beside the bed. Maybe she could just touch Mom's arm.

"No! A proper hug. As in arms around me so I can get my arms around you. Now!" Mom tugged Hannah down.

Hannah held her neck back as far as she could to keep it off Mom's chest. To avoid touching the bandages, she patted at the air around them the best she could.

Mom didn't really have the strength to pull her any closer, so she finally gave up and let Hannah go. It wasn't very satisfying, but at least Hannah knew she hadn't hurt Mom.

When Hannah looked back through the doorway, she saw Mom lower the hand she had been waving and close her eyes.

83

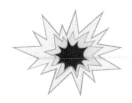

chapter 14
another cancer slam

"Oh, no," Mom said from the computer, where she was checking email.

It was a little odd to see Mom back in the computer chair. She was still wearing loose shirts to make room for the drains, and she still didn't move very fast. But she was back doing many of the things she normally did.

"What, Mom?" Hannah asked.

"You know Matt who went camping with you guys? Apparently last week they had to take him to the emergency room, and he was just diagnosed with lymphoma yesterday. That's terrible!"

Matt? Hannah didn't remember anyone named Matt camping with them. And lymphoma—what was that?

Mom read a little more of the email. "He's already had surgery, and he'll start chemo in a few days."

"Mom, do you only get chemo if you have cancer?"

Mom swiveled in the chair to face Hannah. "Yes, lymphoma is a kind of cancer. Actually I don't know much about it."

M.D. looked up from his trains. "But, nobody named Matt went camping with us. Right, Hannah?"

Hannah shook her head and Mom looked surprised. "Sure he did," Mom said. You know, Jenny's nephew…Matt and Sally—Sally's brother."

"Sally's brother wasn't named Matt. He was Fatty!" Max said.

"Fatty?" Mom looked puzzled.

"Yeah, that's what they called him. *Fatty*. And it was a little weird because he didn't seem to care and he wasn't even fat!" Hannah said.

"*Fatty?*" Mom mused. Then she smiled. "Matt…maybe they call him Matty. That's his nickname. His real name is Matt, or maybe Matthew, and sometimes they call him Matty. Not Fatty."

Hannah turned purple and tried to remember if she had called him Fatty to his face. Mom burst out laughing. It was so good to hear her laughing that Hannah smiled, too. Then she and Max started giggling as well. But, oh, she hoped she hadn't called him Fatty to his face! How embarrassing would that be?!

Mom said, "You know, we really should put together a care package for him and Sally. After Matt's operation, he is going to have to be inside and quiet a lot. We should send him some things to do. And Sally is probably going to get bored at home, especially when she's not the sick one."

"Like the box Rebecca sent us?" Hannah remembered. "That was awesome!"

"Exactly. Think about what sorts of things we can send them. If it were you, what would you guys like?"

That night when Hannah got in the bed, she started thinking about Matty. She knew kids could get cancer, since she had known Rose. But Rose's real home had been very far away, and Rose had been kind of thin and weak-looking. Besides, they hadn't just been camping with Rose. Matty sure hadn't seemed sick, certainly not during the party in the tent. He had told that spooky story that scared Max and her right to the campfire. He'd seemed perfectly well—silly, kind of crazy, just like an ordinary kid. Just like Mom had seemed perfectly well right up until her operation.

Hannah lay in the bed as straight as she could lie. First, she wiggled her toes. They moved easily and nothing hurt. Then she tensed and relaxed her leg muscles. Everything seemed normal. She worked her way all the way up her body, making sure everything moved like it was supposed to and there was no pain.

Just as Hannah was relaxing, thinking there was no way she could have cancer, she remembered Mom had found her cancer by feeling the lump in her breast. Hannah sat up in the darkness. M.D. was whistling softly in his sleep. Only the shadow of the tree outside the window was visible in the darkened room. Its branches swayed around the streets printed on Max's car rug. Outside, the traffic pulsed in a steady rhythm.

Hannah reached for her toes and feet, feeling for lumps, anything that wasn't smooth skin. Slowly she brought her fingers up her legs and to her stomach. She covered her whole body, searching for anything unusual, anything that shouldn't be there.

Everything seemed normal. She found a couple of bug bites and a bruise on her leg from where she'd tripped last week, but other than that, there was only skin, smooth skin.

But there was no way to check her insides. There was no way to be absolutely sure that she really was healthy, that cancer wasn't trying to find a home somewhere in her body.

By the time Hannah lay back down on the cool sheets, sweat had soaked her pajamas. Cancer could come out of nowhere and attack anyone. Would she be its next victim? Tears rolled down her cheeks as the shadowy branches of the tree blew over her bed. Nothing felt safe. It was a dangerous world.

"**h**annah!" The door to their room was flung open and the hall light spilled in. "Honey, what's wrong?" Mom crept to the side of the bunk bed.

Mom touched Hannah's face, "Oh, Sweetie. You're crying. What's the matter?" When Mom cupped her chin, Hannah cried harder.

"Come on down. I can't carry you because of my chest, but come on down. Let's go in the living room."

Suddenly, Dad, his suit coat still on, materialized beside the bed. He dropped his briefcase on the rug and scooped Hannah out of the bed in his arms. Hannah buried her head on his shoulder and sobbed, "I don't want to get cancer. Please, don't let me get cancer."

Dad held her tight and Mom rubbed her back as they walked down the hall into the brightly lit living room. All three of them sat down on the sofa. In between sobs, Hannah told them how she'd checked for cancer, but that she didn't know how to keep it at bay.

"Hannah," Mom said softly. "Are you scared because of Matt?"

Hannah nodded, her head still buried in Dad's shoulder.

Mom filled Dad in, "Matt, from the camping trip, has lymphoma. He's starting chemo next week. We just found out tonight."

Then she turned to Hannah. "It's pretty rare to get cancer. Especially kids."

Mom sat back from Dad and Hannah so she could look Hannah straight in the eye. "Cancer is a big term for cells that aren't normal. Sometimes cells in your body mutate, or change, and then those changed cells keep dividing. For some reason, cancer cells divide more quickly than normal cells, so one of the problems with cancer cells is that there are a lot of them quickly. When that happens, they start crowding out normal cells.

"There are lots of different kinds of cancer. And cancers in different parts of your body can act differently," Mom went on in a calm voice. "It's pretty confusing. Doctors and scientists have figured out some things that cause many different kinds of cancer. They haven't figured out the entire list of causes for all cancers, but there are certain risk factors that make it more likely a person will get cancer."

Hannah looked puzzled. "Like what?" she asked.

Mom explained further. "Like, we know that smoking can cause lung cancer and sunburns can cause skin cancer. That doesn't mean that everyone who gets a sunburn will get skin cancer, but it does mean that if you get a sunburn, you are at a higher risk for skin cancer."

"What makes you at a higher risk for breast cancer?" Hannah wanted to know.

Mom thought a minute. "Being an older woman increases the likelihood that you might get breast cancer. Having a mom or a grandmom who has had it increases your risk. Obesity, or being too heavy, and consuming too much alcohol can both be factors in whether you get breast cancer."

"But, Mom," Hannah protested, "you're not any of those things—old or fat. And Gram hasn't had breast cancer, has she? Do you drink too much?" Hannah demanded.

"No," Mom shook her head, "Gram hasn't had cancer, and I don't drink too much, at least not very often!" Hannah could see Dad smiling at Mom over Hannah's head. "Those factors don't mean you are going to get cancer, but when scientists have looked at all the people who have gotten diagnosed with breast cancer, many, but not all, of them have one or more of those factors."

Mom continued, "There's not something specific that the doctors can point to that caused my cancer. But, scientists also think that certain factors in our environment, the places where we live and work, might cause some cancer. Lots of scientists are doing all kinds of research and testing to better understand what these things might be.

"Kids don't get cancer very often because it takes a long time for whatever it is that is bad in the environment to build up enough in their bodies to cause the cells to change. Generally kids just haven't lived long enough for that to happen."

When Mom paused, Hannah raised her head up from Dad's shoulder. When she tried to wipe the big wet patch on his jacket away with her tissue, he just shrugged his shoulder and smiled. "It's OK It'll dry."

Hannah faced Mom. "But then, why does Matty have it? He's just a year older than me."

Mom leaned back on the arm of the sofa and sighed. "We just don't know. Doctors and scientists are working hard to try to figure it out. Some people are probably born with some cells already mutated but they don't know it. Until those people have some symptoms of the disease, there is no reason to think that they have cancer. Matt's leg hurt a lot. That's how they knew something was wrong. My symptom was the lump in my breast. Cancer can be in your body for a long time before it causes any symptoms."

Dad rubbed Hannah's head. He said reassuringly, "Hannah, we can't promise you won't get cancer. But the chance that you will get it is pretty slim."

"And another thing," Mom added, "part of the reason you get a check-up every year is so the doctor can see if any part of your body has changed in a way that might be suspicious. The best thing we can do to prevent cancer is to get regular check-ups and be as healthy as we can at home. Why do you think I make you eat fruits and vegetables at every meal? It's not only because I'm mean!" Mom smiled a little.

Then Mom continued, "You know, when I first learned I had cancer, I was really scared, first just about cancer in general and then that it might come back. And it might. But then I realized I don't have any control over whether it comes back or not. But there are some things I do have control over—like eating as healthily as I can and getting my arms strong again from the surgery. That's why I have been doing my arm exercises so much." Mom stretched her arm as far up over her head as she could to demonstrate.

Hannah smiled. Mom did look pretty silly when she flattened herself up against the wall and tried to reach for the ceiling. She couldn't get very far right now, but when she first got home from the hospital, Mom had gotten Dad to draw a line on the wall with a pencil and every day she kept trying to reach it. She'd said that when she could do that, she was going to erase that line and get Dad to draw another one higher up.

When Dad had drawn the first line, right when Mom had come home from the hospital, Mom could barely lift her arm at all. Max had been fascinated watching Dad drawing on the wall. Mom had given Max her most polished evil eye. "You are not to draw on the wall. Do you understand? You can draw on paper or on your easel, but not on the wall." Just as Max had started to protest, Mom held up her hand to stop him. "When you have your own apartment, then you can draw all over your very own wall, but not on ours. Get it?" Max had nodded reluctantly, disappointed.

Now, though, Dad opened up one of his arms to make room for Mom, and she moved beside him, nestling her head in the wet patch on Dad's shoulder. Hannah rested her head back on Mom's collarbone. The three of them formed a triangle.

Mom rubbed Hannah's arms. "It's going to be fine, Hannah. I'm not saying it will exactly be like it was. But it's going to be fine."

They sat like that a long time, and Hannah wanted to believe her so badly.

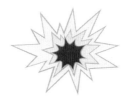

chapter 15
mornings

h annah studied her hair in the bathroom mirror. Why had she agreed to get it cut again? She'd never have Lydia's long locks at the rate she was going.

Last spring, she'd grown it out for an organization that gives wigs to people who lose their hair from chemo. (She thought it was ironic that she did this before they even knew about Mom's cancer.) By the time they had lopped off the ten inches required for a donation, her hair had been pretty short, right at her chin. At the time, she had liked it, especially since her bangs were finally grown out, but now she really wanted to be able to put it in a ponytail.

Just before the diagnosis, though, Mom asked if Hannah wanted to get it cut again. Stupidly, she'd said yes. Why did she do that? Now, even a few months later, no matter how she tried to style it, it just wouldn't stay back.

While Hannah was muttering to herself about her hair, Max was weighing himself on the scale. He had figured out if he gripped the towel bar while he weighed, he could lose a pound or two. Now he was trying to see if he could make himself heavier without picking anything up. He took a flying leap onto the scale.

Mom turned off the shower and reached for her towel. Max stopped his scale tricks and stared at her with his head tilted.

"Mommy, when they finish putting your fake boobs on, will you be as wobbly as you were before?"

Mom burst out laughing. "Max-buddy," she replied, "thanks to the magic of fake boobs, I will never be as wobbly as I was before. Wobblier than I am now, but never as wobbly as before!"

Hannah studied Mom's chest in the bathroom mirror so Mom wouldn't know she was staring. There were two thin lines, scars Hannah assumed, on very small mounds where Mom's breasts used to be. The mounds were round like small, hard balls. Not soft like her breasts had been before the operation.

There wasn't any color there either. Mom said that the pink circle part of a breast was called an areola and the nipple was in the middle of the areola. The doctor would tattoo on an areola and later, if Mom wanted him to, he could add a fake nipple, too.

Mom finished drying off with the towel, very carefully patting around her chest and under her arms. When she noticed both of them staring at her, Mom looked down at her chest. "They're kind of weird looking, don't you think? Kind of like skin-colored tennis balls. Do you guys want to feel them?"

With her towel wrapped around her waist, she squatted down, and both Hannah and Max reached over to feel where the expanders, a.k.a. water balloons, were. It was very weird, like feeling a smooth, round ball under Mom's skin.

Then Mom pointed to a bump on the edge of the expander on her chest. "That's called a port. That's where they stick the needle to put more fluid in. The fluid is what makes my skin and muscle stretch."

"Ohh, does it hurt?" Max's eyes filled with sympathy.

"No, I don't have any feeling where the port is. I can feel something pushing in but it doesn't hurt." Mom pulled her robe around her shoulders.

"Mommy, do you slosh around with all that water in your chest?" Max asked.

Mom gave her shoulders a little shake and grinned. "I don't hear anything. Do you?"

Max got her to shake again and listened carefully. He shook his head sadly.

"Just a couple more expansions," Mom said, "and then I'll be done." That was good news. Mom hated the expansion sessions because she felt like her eyeballs were being stretched out.

"Then you'll get your fake boobs?" Max asked.

"Well, they have to wait for about eight weeks after I finish chemo before they can do that. So, I'll probably get them just before you guys get out of school in June."

"That's a long time to have tennis balls stuck to your chest," Max said.

Mom agreed. "Well, that's just the way it is. Nothing I can do about it." She put on one of her shirts that buttoned in front. She still couldn't raise her hands over her head very well.

"When will you get your tattoo?" Hannah asked curiously.

"Tattoo?" Max looked up interestedly. "Can you pick what you want for a tattoo?"

Mom looked puzzled.

"You know, like a leopard...or a pretty butterfly maybe?" Max added hopefully.

Mom started laughing again. "No, Buddy. I'm going to have nice pink circles there. That's all!"

"But..." Max looked dejected over this bit of news.

"When you are all grown up, you can get a leopard tattoo if you want, but pink circles are as far into the world of tattoos as I am venturing!" Mom said firmly.

"Everything fun is only when I'm all growed up!" Max sighed.

When Mom had her shirt on, Hannah really couldn't tell that anything was different. Hannah glanced down at her own chest, which was flat. Why Mom would want to go to all that trouble to have a fake chest? She could have just left things as they were after the surgery and stayed flat.

Right before Mom's mastectomy, Hannah had overheard Mom tell a friend that she had already nursed her kids, so she wasn't going to need her breasts any more. If that were true, then why did Mom want the implants? Hannah couldn't figure out why anyone would volunteer to get stuck with a needle for something she wasn't going to need again. It didn't make any sense to her, but then grownups frequently didn't make sense to Hannah, so this wasn't a new thought.

W hen Hannah got up the next morning, Max was curled up in Mom and Dad's bed with Mom. "Mommy, will you please read me a book?" he begged in his cutest voice. Hannah hated that voice. Whenever he used it, she automatically wanted to say "no" to whatever he was asking.

"I can't read you a book right now!" Mom protested as she swung her legs over Max's snuggled-up bump.

"Why not?"

"Because it's a school morning, and I have to get up and get my shower and then we have to get you ready for school. That's why. Now come on. We have to get up."

"OK, Mommy. But after you get your strong medicine and you get bald, then you won't have to wash your hair in the morning. Then you will have lots of time, even in the mornings, and you can read me books in bed, OK? That will be nice."

"Well, we'll see…" was all Mom would promise as she got in the shower.

Hannah burst into the bathroom just as Mom was climbing out of the shower, wrapping a towel around herself and rubbing her hair dry. "Mom, I need you to sign my homework sheet. And here's my permission slip for our field trip to the Metropolitan Museum. I need five dollars for it. They need chaperones. Can you go with us?" Hannah's words came out all in a rush.

Mom pulled the towel tight before saying, "Whoa, Missy. You know you're supposed to unpack your backpack the night before, put your lunchbox in the kitchen, and give me anything that needs signing. You'll have to put it on the kitchen counter. If I can get to it before we leave for school, I will. Where's your lunchbox?"

"But, Mom! I need that stuff today. Ms. Calde said we might not be able to go if I don't turn in my money today. And if you want to chaperone, she needs to know that today too! Please?" Hannah begged with her eyes. Occasionally, Mom could be won over by tears.

"Where's your lunchbox?" Mom repeated. "If it wasn't in the kitchen last night, you'll have to make your own lunch," she said trying to go around Hannah, who was standing in the middle of the bathroom doorway.

Dad intervened, his face lathered white with shaving cream. "Look, Hannah, if you put the stuff on the kitchen counter, Mom will probably have time to get to it this morning. If you continue standing here blocking the door, you're just wasting everyone's time."

Hannah turned her eyes up at him. "But, I really want Mom to chaperone, and I have to tell Ms. Calde today," she begged desperately.

It worked, and Dad melted. He looked at Mom, "Liz, can you?"

Mom sighed. "I have to check the calendar and see when the trip is. Hannah, I just can't promise. Chemo will start soon, and I don't think I'm going to feel that great. But I'll check the calendar. Still," Mom continued, "you need to unpack the night before. You know that. Otherwise there isn't time to do all this in the morning. Now, go put your stuff on the counter! And," Mom added in a very exasperated tone, "where is your lunchbox?!"

"Mommy, you haven't been on one of my trips either!" M.D. started to whine.

Mom cut him off quickly as she threw her clothes on. "That's because your class hasn't been on any trips. I can't go on a trip that hasn't happened. Go get your bed made up!"

In the kitchen, Mom looked at the calendar on the fridge. The days leading up to her surgery were covered with ink from all of her appointments and tests she had had. Then there was a long string of blank days—all of the time it would take her to recover from surgery, Hannah guessed. Now that they were past the empty squares on the calendar, ink once again was beginning to fill the blocks.

Mom compared the date of the trip with a square on the calendar. "Oh, Hannah. My first oncologist appointment is that day. I can't change it. I'm sorry."

Hannah's eyes filled up with real tears then.

Mom looked over at her and then wrapped her arm around Hannah's shoulder. "Oh, Sweetie. I promise before this year is out, I will go on a trip with you—and you, too," she nodded at Max. "But it probably won't happen until spring. I know the teachers like to give all the parents a chance to go on one of the trips. I'll just take my turn later in the year. It'll be all right. You'll see."

Then Mom turned her attention to the mound of paperwork Hannah had left on the counter. "If you'll go get my wallet, I'll give you money for your trip."

"Can't you change your appointment?" Hannah begged.

"No, I can't. I need to start on chemo as soon as possible, and with Thanksgiving coming up, there isn't a lot of time. Now, where's my wallet? And where is your lunchbox?"

Max yelped, "I'll get your wallet, Mommy!" while Hannah wiped her eyes with the back of her hand. Nothing was normal and it didn't seem like anything ever would be again.

Mom pushed the peanut butter and bread in Hannah's direction on the counter, and Dad started pulling cereal bowls out of the cabinet.

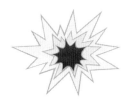

chapter 16
reinstated vacation

annah answered the phone after school one day. "Hello?" It was Aunt Kath. Hannah handed the phone to Mom.

"Hi, Kath!" Mom said cheerfully, matching Aunt Kath's perpetual enthusiasm.

While Hannah unpacked her backpack (this time when she was supposed to), she heard Mom say that she was feeling much better and was moving around pretty well. Just then life improved dramatically.

"Oh, we're definitely still planning to come. Yeah, by that point, it will have been five weeks since the surgery. Besides, we're all really ready to get out of the city, and I know Hannah would kill me if we had to miss seeing you guys!"

Hannah didn't hear anything else while it all registered. They weren't going to miss their Thanksgiving trip after all! Everything had been on hold to see how Mom felt after surgery. But now it sounded like in a week or so they would get to see Will, Hugh, and Jimmy! Yeah!

When Hannah focused again, Mom was saying, "Well, I was thinking of taking the kids out of school for a couple of days. That way we'll miss some traffic and have a good long break. John might ride up with us, even if he does have to work once we're there." Dad often had to work during vacations. "Or, he can just take the train later in the week," Mom added.

There was a pause on Mom's side of the conversation. Then, "We're looking forward to it, too. Let's talk over the weekend to confirm plans."

When she hung up the phone, Mom saw Hannah grinning. Mom returned the smile and said, "I told you life as we know it isn't completely over!"

"Over? What's over? Your cansker?" Max asked as he drove his big yellow truck into the living room and over Hannah's foot.

"...*cer*. Can*cer*." Hannah muttered at him for the millionth time hopping around, holding her toe. Then she beamed, poised to tell him the good news. "No! Mom's cancer isn't over!"

Mom started laughing, "Well, you don't have to say that so cheerfully!" she said.

"Uhh, I mean, yes, we hope her cancer's over. But, no, she's not finished. She still has to have chemo..." Hannah trailed off, suddenly feeling very confused.

"I'm teasing, Hannah. You can tell him the news."

Max cocked his head to the side. "What news, Hannah?"

"We get to go to Will, Hugh, and Jimmy's for Thanks-giving!" Hannah shouted. Max started jumping up and down. Hannah grabbed his hands, and they did huge kicks all around the living room in their excitement.

Mom shook her head at them and turned to go into the kitchen to heat up some dinner. "Do you want leftover lasagna or chick...ooh! Ow!" Hannah and Max heard a huge thud and the sound of plastic scraping the kitchen floor.

When they looked over at Mom, she was on all fours on the ground, and the big yellow truck had skidded to a stop in front of the refrigerator. "Mom, are you OK?" Hannah asked, running over to her.

"I just tripped on that..." Mom pointed to Max's truck and then shifted so she was sitting. "Ohhh, it hurts. Probably just a bruise, but whew! This is painful," Mom said, gently massaging the lump beginning to poke up on her leg.

"I will get the boo-boo pack for you," Max announced, shoving the truck out of the way to retrieve the icepack from the freezer.

He plopped the boo-boo pack down next to Mom's leg and then plopped himself into her lap. "Are we really going to New Hampshire for Thanksgiving, Mommy?"

Mom raised her eyebrows and pursed her lips, drawing in a quick breath. She nodded, her lips pressed together tightly, while holding the icepack to her bruise.

"Can we go camping there? Can we have another party in the tent?" Max begged.

"Should we call Dad?" Hannah asked, pointing to Mom's leg.

Mom lifted up the icepack. The lump was already very purple. "No, I'll be fine. It just hurts. Max, how many times have I told you not to leave your toys in the middle of the kitchen floor? This is why," she said gesturing at her bruise. "Thank goodness I didn't hit my chest!"

103

"Why? Would your water balloons pop?" Max wanted to know.

Mom nodded. "Maybe. I don't know."

While Hannah looked worriedly at Mom's chest, which suddenly seemed very fragile, Max asked delightedly, "Would water come squirting out of you?"

"Not out of me, but out of the expanders. Then I'd have to have more put in. Yuck!"

"More water or more balloons?" Max asked.

Mom looked down at Max both fondly and with a little irritation. "Both, probably. And I definitely don't want more surgery. Otherwise we won't get to go away for Thanksgiving!"

Max and Hannah started marking off the days until the Thanksgiving trip on the kitchen calendar. They had circled the day they were leaving in red. Mom was going to get them out of school at noon on the Tuesday before Thanksgiving.

e ven though it was only about a week away, the days felt like they had slowed to a crawl, and it didn't help that this November was a rainy month. There wasn't much playing in the park after school.

Hannah couldn't help but notice the writing on the square the day after they got back. The trip to the Met and Mom's first oncologist's appointment. The oncologist was the doctor who would give her the chemotherapy. He was the one who was going to make Mom lose her hair and be so sick. How could his name be written on her calendar so innocently? As far as Hannah was concerned, that day should be marked with the big, black X.

One evening, Mom saw Hannah pretend to rub out that date on the calendar. Mom smiled a little. "Yeah, I'm not looking forward to that day either." Then she shrugged. "But, in a way, it's good. The sooner I start, the sooner I'll be done. And the sooner I start, the sooner we can zap any renegade cancer cells!"

Then Mom sighed. "It sure would be nice to go back a year ago, when we didn't even know about all of this, wouldn't it? But then we'd have it all in front of us, even if we didn't know it. So I suppose that really wouldn't be so good."

Mom shook off her mood and said, "Hannah, would you check the computer? I think there's an email for you."

An email for her? Almost unheard of! When Hannah pulled it up on the computer, she saw Will had written, asking if they wanted to camp out in the backyard. If so, he said, she and Max needed to bring their sleeping bags.

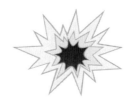

chapter 17
mr. trump

ms. Calde flickered the lights to get the class's
attention. "I know no one wants to think about
the history project over Thanksgiving, but I just
want to remind you that if you're staying here in the city, it
might be a good time to visit your individual sites."

Everyone groaned.

"I know," Ms. Calde added, "that you aren't going to
make your presentations until spring, but if you visit your site
in a couple of seasons, I guarantee you'll see something
different every time. It will make for a richer report."

"Rich?" Scottie snickered. "Is anyone researching Trump
Plaza?"

Ms. Calde smiled into the sea of giggles. "Even Trump
Plaza looks different at different times of the year," she said.
"The holiday decorations there in December are stereotypical
New York excess and certainly define one aspect of modern
New York. Part of your job on your project is to figure out
what your individual sites tell us about your group's time
period in the city's history."

"Huh?" Carl said, confused.

Lydia leaned out into the aisle and twisted around to address Carl. "She means that the decorations for Trump Plaza cost a lot of money, like a lot of things in the city. The fact that Mr. Trump puts them up means he's rich, which is what a lot of people think all New Yorkers are." Lydia swished her ponytail in a high arc as she straightened herself back in her seat.

"Well, I'm not rich!" Carl protested.

"That's what a stereotype is," Ms. Calde nodded. "Thinking everyone in a certain group is the same. Some people here in the city are wealthy and do spend a lot of money on things that get photographed frequently, like buildings, decorations, and clothes. Those photographs are often all that other people know of New York. So they think that everyone in New York lives that way."

"That's stupid," Carl muttered. "I'm not rich, and I've lived in New York my whole life. I sure wish I was, though!"

Mary raised her hand tentatively. "Or, television shows. My aunt went to China, and some people there thought everyone in the United States lived on a plantation because of a TV show they had seen."

Ms. Calde nodded. "Exactly. We all form stereotypes about people or places we don't know. The only way to break them is to get to know the people being stereotyped for who they really are. If all you've ever seen of the United States is plantations, then that's where you think everyone in the U.S. lives. If all you've ever seen of New York is the Trump Plaza decorated at Christmas time, then that's what you think all of New York looks like. The way we change those perceptions is to show other sides of ourselves. The way we avoid stereotyping other people is to look for more than one side to them."

Ms. Calde paused and looked around the room. She added, "Part of the purpose of the history project is to figure out if there is a stereotype of your time period. If so, then you have to decide whether or not it is accurate. If not, what is the real story?"

Hannah rubbed her forehead tiredly. She really had to get busy learning something, anything, about Thomas Paine and his park. Maybe Mom could take her down there before they left on their Thanksgiving trip.

S cottie banged his hand down on the lunch table a couple of times. "That's a good one!" he chortled. "What about you, Hannah?"

"What about me what?" Hannah asked, fishing her yogurt out of her lunch box.

"What would you buy if you were rich? Sam wants a cook. He's tired of eating burned chicken nuggets!"

"And pizza. I'm really, really sick of pizza," Sam sighed.

Lydia tilted her head towards their end of the table. "You should just learn to cook. Then you could make yourself whatever you like." She blinked her eyes several times.

Sam shrugged and went back to his peanut butter.

Mary said, "I'd buy a car. Whenever my sister and I want to go somewhere, my parents don't want to rent a car." Mary chewed thoughtfully on her tuna sandwich. Then she added, "And a garage space nearby. I don't think my mom would be too excited about parking a car on the street."

Hannah busied herself making a pile of her lunch garbage. If she could really, truly buy anything she wanted, she would buy a bigger apartment so she could have her own room.

Carl mumbled through a mouthful of potato chips, "I'd buy a flat screen TV. Our TV is so old that the picture is kind of blurry!"

Hannah mentally decorated her very own room. Turquoise walls, a white bed, and crisp new sheets—oh, and a door that shut firmly so Max couldn't come in.

"Hannah?" Scottie asked again. "What would you buy?"

"Oh, I don't know…," Hannah mused.

Lydia jumped in. "Well, I'd buy a day at the spa. A massage and a facial would feel so good! And my nails sure could use some attention." Lydia waved her perfectly polished fingertips over the table for everyone to see.

Mary prompted Hannah again. "What do you want?"

Lydia pursed her lips tightly together when no one commented on her wish.

"I don't know," Hannah repeated. "My own room would be nice, I guess."

"Oh yeah!" Heads bobbed up and down the table. Almost everyone in Hannah's class had to share a room with a sibling.

"Well, I don't need my own room," Lydia announced. "I don't have to share my room with anyone."

Hannah collected her garbage as the whistle blew signaling the end of lunch. Having her own room was almost unfathomable.

Suddenly, two arms wound around her waist. Max grinned up at her. "Hi, Hannah!" he said as he squeezed.

"Max! Come find your line partner!" Max's teacher gestured for him. Hannah returned the hug before unraveling Max's hands and giving him a little push back towards his teacher. When Max got back to the line, he turned and waved both hands vigorously, grinning like the silly four-year-old he was.

"'Bye, Max! I'll see you later!" Hannah called and waved back.

Then she went back to her own thoughts. "I do want my own room, but I'm glad I have a brother. Most of the time, anyway. Lydia must get awfully lonely with no other kids in her apartment."

She glanced at Max's class disappearing up the stairs. "I wonder if Max is glad to have a sister?"

"So which would you choose?"

Hannah jerked her head up, startled, "Huh?" she said, almost spitting in Mary's face.

Hannah flushed red. "Sorry," she murmured, wiping her mouth with the back of her hand.

Mary giggled. "No problem." Then she asked again, "Which would you choose, having your own room, but no Max at all, or having a brother but having to share a room with him?"

Hannah's mouth fell open. "How did you know what I was thinking?" she gasped.

"You were thinking out loud," Mary smiled.

Hannah rubbed her chin with her thumb and forefinger thoughtfully. "I don't know. I guess I'd just keep on sharing with Max, even if he does drive me crazy sometimes."

Mary nodded. "My sister's older than me. She can be so bossy sometimes. But sometimes she's a lot of fun. I'd miss her."

Scottie, who was hovering nearby, burst out laughing. "No, you wouldn't! How could you miss her? She wouldn't have ever been there for you to miss!"

Hannah looked at Mary and then started giggling, too. "He's right. You can't miss someone who doesn't exist!"

The hurt look on Mary's face disappeared as she dropped the rest of her trash into the garbage can. She grinned at them. "I think I'll just stick to buying a car…when I'm rich, that is!

"By the way," Mary said quietly to Hannah. "It's easy to see that Max is pretty glad to have a sister."

Hannah smiled and looked back at the stairs Max's class had climbed. She nodded slowly. "Thanks, Mary. That's awfully nice."

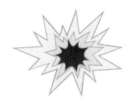

chapter 18
communication rift

"What's it like?" Will asked as the campfire slowly died out.

"What's what like?" Hannah said, using a stick to poke at the few red flecks still winking in the fire pit. They had set the tent up Thanksgiving afternoon, but the grownups said that the weather looked too iffy to stay out all night. None of the kids were too happy about it, but as a compromise, they'd all toasted marshmallows over a campfire in the backyard.

"You know," Will said, not really looking at her.

"What are you talking about?" Hannah asked him. Being evasive wasn't usually Will's style.

"You know," he repeated, reaching into the nearly empty marshmallow bag. "With your mom and all..."

"What's what like with my mom?" Hannah asked, puzzled. If she lifted the stick up slowly enough, when she tipped it there was a small soot shower. "She's just Mom. I mean she had the surgery and she's still pretty sore. But mostly she acts normal, just like any mom."

"No," Will mumbled through a mouthful of raw marshmallow. "I mean, with her going to die and everything."

"Die? She's not going to die! Who said she was going to die?" Hannah fixed her most piercing stare right onto Will until he had no choice but to look back at her.

He swallowed the lump of marshmallow in his mouth and then licked his lips.

"Who, Will? Who said that?" Hannah demanded.

"Well, no one's said she's going to die specifically. But she does have cancer and cancer generally means you're gonna die. Cancer kills people."

The dying embers popped in the ensuing silence. Then Hannah snapped, "Everyone dies, Will. Everyone. So, yeah, my mom's going to die. So is yours. But Mom's not going to die from breast cancer. She's just not. They got all the cancer with the surgery.

Well," Hannah corrected herself slightly, "they're pretty sure did they did anyway."

"So why's she gonna have chemo? Chemo means you're really sick, dying sick," Will retorted, returning Hannah's glare.

"Chemo makes you really sick. It doesn't necessarily mean you already are! She's going to have chemo in case they didn't get it all. It's supposed to kill any cancer cells that might still be there."

Hannah punched at the embers a few more times and then threw her stick down. "I'm going to go find Max," she said, marching off towards the house.

"Hey, Hannah," Will turned towards Hannah. "Don't be mad. I'm sorry. I just…I just…well, I just know cancer's really bad. I'm really sorry," he finished lamely.

"Sorry cancer's bad or sorry you said something stupid?" Hannah snarled.

As she stormed into the house, Hannah exploded over her shoulder, "Cancer is bad, but that doesn't mean everyone has to die from it. And even if Mom was dying, which she's not, it wouldn't be any of your business!"

Mom and Aunt Kath were having a glass of wine by the fireplace. Hannah threw off her coat and barked at them, louder than she meant to, "Where's Max?"

Mom raised her eyebrows and looked over the top of her glasses. "Want to try that again?"

"Sorry," Hannah took a deep breath. "Do you know where Max is?"

"Dad and Uncle Jeff took Max and Hugh upstairs to put them in the bathtub. I'm assuming that's where they still are," Mom said. She eyed Hannah, concerned. "Is everything OK? Where's Will?" Mom added.

"Still out there." Hannah jerked her thumb towards the door.

"Did he do something?" Aunt Kath wanted to know.

Hannah shook her head and headed up the stairs. "I'm going to get my shower."

When she got to the top, she heard the back door slam.

"Will," Aunt Kath was asking, "is everything OK?"

"Yeah," Will answered shortly.

"I mean with Hannah."

"Yeah, I guess. I asked her a question, and she got mad. Dad said I'll never really understand girls, and, boy, is he ever right! And she's not even my girlfriend; she's just my cousin!"

Mom and Aunt Kath chuckled. Hannah snatched her towel from the back of the door.

That night, while lying on the air mattress, listening to Max's nighttime whistle, Hannah was still fuming.

What gave Will the right to say Mom was dying? But, maybe, Mom was. Mom had been crying in the living room one night not too long ago when Hannah got up to go to the bathroom. Maybe Mom and Dad had told Aunt Kath and Uncle Jeff that she was dying, but not told her and Max. Hannah knew parents sometimes tell their own kids the important stuff last. And cancer was really bad, without a doubt. The doctors had had to cut off part of Mom to get rid of it. So, maybe Mom *was* dying.

Strange shadows crept along the ceiling while Max whistled away. If Mom was dying, then Hannah was really mad at Mom for not telling her. But that didn't absolve Will's stupid comments. Wasn't there anywhere she could go without being reminded of breast cancer? Cancer was becoming her whole life!

Hannah rolled over and squeezed her eyes shut. Mom was not dying, Hannah told herself. Some parents tell their kids last, but not her parents. She reminded herself that they had told her and Max about the cancer when they first got the diagnosis, before they told anyone else. She knew Mom and Dad would tell them if Mom was really dying.

Besides, why would Mom get chemo if she were really dying? Chemo sounded so bad, it might make you die, particularly if you were already really sick. Hannah didn't think they'd give it to someone who was already really sick.

No, Mom couldn't be dying—she was getting ready to live! Yes, that was it! Getting ready to live. That would make a good line a poem, Hannah thought. Dad's vote on it would be "Cheesy!" But it would still be a good line.

When she released her eyes, she saw that snow had started falling. She snuggled closer to Max under the blanket and finally stopped thinking. She dreamed of drifts of white marshmallows.

m ax's joyful shrieks woke Hannah up the next morning. "Hannah! Look! It's snowing!"

Hannah crawled off the mattress, keeping her blanket wrapped tightly around her and went to the window. It must have snowed all night.

"Boy, am I glad Mom and Dad said no camping! Look at the tent!" The tent Dad had helped Uncle Jeff pitch in the backyard yesterday was almost buried under snow. The tops of the tent poles were barely visible in the clouds of white. "Wow!"

Hugh and Jimmy came flying down the stairs. "Hurry, get your snow pants on! Let's go out before breakfast!" Hugh urged as he threw open a closet and rummaged around.

"No snow pants here, Mom!" Hugh yelled up the stairs.

Aunt Kath came down the stairs a little more slowly than the boys had, carrying a coffee mug in her hands. "Hi, guys!" she said brightly to Hannah and Max. "Did you see what the weatherman sent our way? Hannah, did you guys bring your snow pants? Do you want to get them and go out before breakfast?"

Max went tearing towards the room Mom and Dad were using. Mom pulled the door open just as Max was about to push on it. Max fell flat on his face. That cracked Hugh and Jimmy up, and they chortled and pointed at Max lying there on the floor.

Mom carefully stepped over Max. She was carrying a wad of outdoor clothes and smiling a big smile. She handed Hannah the clothing bundle. "Somehow, I thought you'd want these." Max scrambled up to get his snow pants.

When they were all layered up and ready to go, Aunt Kath announced that she wanted to take a picture.

"Where's Will?" Aunt Kath asked as she tried to assemble them into an entity worthy of a photograph.

"Jeff," she shouted up the stairs, "is Will up there? Send him down to get in the picture before going out in the snow."

Jimmy and Max wriggled in their layers while they waited for Will to come down. Sweat dripped down Hannah's back. "Mom! I'm hot!" she complained

"Will!" Aunt Kath called again. "Will, come on..."

Uncle Jeff appeared at the top of the stairs. "He's in his room, but he says he doesn't want to go out."

When Aunt Kath started to protest, Uncle Jeff just shrugged.

Hannah wiped more sweat off her face.

"Ok, then," Aunt Kath said after a pause and turned back to the mob of kids. With the camera up to her eye, she announced, "Picture time!"

h annah thought the rest of the weekend was pretty weird. Will did his own thing, which left her to hang out with the littler guys. Even when they'd all watched a movie, Will had stayed upstairs reading a book or playing on the computer.

At one point, Hugh, Max, and Hannah tunneled their way through the snow into the tent and crawled in. But when the little kids started telling stupid four-and-five-year-old jokes, Hannah left them snorting with laughter and dug her way out of the tent.

All that snow sure was pretty. So white and fresh. Hannah aimlessly began to pack snow and then realized her pile of snowballs was actually the beginnings of a pretty good wall. Just as it got tall enough so she could barely see over it, the back door opened and Jimmy hurtled out.

"Handy, Handy," he yelped, using his nickname for her, slamming into the wall like a flying missile.

He hit full-force, and the whole wall came crumbling down.

"Kind of the opposite of Humpty-Dumpty," Hannah thought grumpily kicking at the ruins and picking Jimmy up from the snow. "Jimmy stayed whole and my wall fell down."

"Oh, Hannah, I'm so sorry," Aunt Kath said, coming up behind them. "He got out the door before I had my coat on. Here, we'll help you build another one." Aunt Kath started making a snowball.

"Oh, it's OK," Hannah said. "I was just fooling around. I'm pretty cold. I think I'll go inside."

Aunt Kath nodded. "Will's in there. Your mom feels like getting out a bit, so she and your dad are going to try out our snowshoes. You could use Hugh's, and you and Will could go, too."

"Maybe," Hannah mumbled, heading for the back steps. She knew Will wouldn't go snowshoeing, at least not with her. She wasn't at all sorry that they were going home the next day.

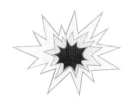

chapter 19
christmas preparations

fter the Thanksgiving holiday, the number of squares on the calendar that had buffered Mom from her oncologist appointment dwindled rapidly. Max and Hannah kept marking off the days, this time counting down to Christmas and, in the process, Mom's appointment.

"Well," Mom said at dinner the night after her doctor's appointment, "at least now I know when I start, next Thursday. That's settled." Mom had thrown her shoulders back and was sitting very straight, but her eyes looked a little tired and more than a bit red.

"Did you go by yourself?" Hannah asked.

"No, Dad came, too." When Max started looking around, Mom added, "Then Dad went back to work. He'll be home later."

"Now will you be bald?" Max wanted to know.

Mom stretched her neck to the side and rolled her shoulders in circles. "Yeah, once they put that medicine in me, it's curtains for my hair."

"Curtains? They give you curtains to wear instead of your hair? Are they special cansker curtains?" Max looked up from his dinner, very interested.

"Cancer." Hannah said for the millionth time, rolling her eyes.

At the same time, Mom said, "Close," with a laugh.

"Close, but no cigar," Hannah sniffed. "No, Silly. Curtains means that's it for Mom's hair. Like in the show *Mary Poppins*, the curtains go down at the end of the show and that's it. Show's over. After the first chemo, Mom's hair is over, done, finished." Hannah added with a dramatic flair.

Max thought about this for a minute, with his forkful of casserole paused mid-way to his mouth. "But in *Mary Poppins*, the curtain went down and we got to get a drink. And then after we finished our drinks, the curtain came back up, and there was more show."

"Intermission," Mom broke in. "That's when we got the drink. The curtain did come back up didn't it? That's sort of like my hair. My hair will take a little intermission and then it'll come back. Just like the show. Anyway, I was thinking when the time comes for it to fall out, do you guys want to give me a haircut?"

Max dropped his fork in his excitement. "Me cut your hair, Mommy?" he asked incredulously.

"Hey! Me, too!" Hannah jumped in.

"Both of you," Mom said, bending over to pick up a wayward pea with her napkin. "We'll have a haircutting party. After all, it's going to fall out anyway. We might as well have some fun with it. One of my email friends let her kids cut her hair. That's where I got the idea."

Mom had some friends she had met on email, all of whom had had to deal with breast cancer. She had actually never met most of them in person, but she seemed to know a lot about them. Hannah wondered if they knew as much about her.

"When?" Max got right down to business. "When are we going to give you a haircut?" He got up from the table and went straight over to the calendar on the refrigerator.

"Let's see," Mom said, following him to look at the squares on the calendar. "I won't actually lose my hair until about time for the second round of chemo, which will be here," and Mom pointed at a date.

"But, the thing is, I don't want my hair to fall out on my pillow or in the shower. I don't think I would like that. I want you guys to cut it before it's supposed to fall out." She scrutinized the calendar carefully. "Maybe here?" She pointed to a square.

"When is that? How many days before we get to cut your hair?" Max demanded.

Mom nodded at the calendar, twirling a strand of hair around her finger. "Yeah, that should be about right. Uh, let's see…" she turned back to Max. "That's in about two weeks. Not tomorrow. Not the next Friday, but the next one. OK?"

Max's face fell. "That's a lot of Fridays," he complained.

"Well, we have lots to do in all those Fridays!" Mom said. "We have to start getting ready for Christmas!"

t was hard to believe that it was already time to get ready for Christmas. But it also felt like they had been waiting forever. At least cancer wasn't keeping Christmas from coming.

Mom was worried that after chemo she might not have a lot of energy to put up all the decorations, so she wanted to get them up before her start date. She and Dad had the same argument every year about Christmas decorations. She always wanted to put them up the first few days of December and take them down before New Year's Day. Dad always wanted to wait and put them up in the middle of December and then take them down after Epiphany, the celebration of the arrival of the three wise men on January 6th. Mom won every year, but this year Dad didn't even give his argument a token try.

That Saturday, Dad got the boxes down from the top of the closet because Mom still wasn't supposed to lift anything. Then he and Max went to the corner to buy a Christmas tree.

Getting a tree in the city was pretty cool, Hannah thought. Foresters came from faraway places, like Maine and Canada, to sell their trees on the same street corners every year. They lived in their trucks from Thanksgiving weekend until Christmas Eve, making themselves right at home by firing up camping stoves and lighting bonfires near their tree displays. Christmas Eve night, after they'd sold their last tree, some of them drove all night to get back to their families for Christmas.

The summer before, when the Bennetts were in Maine, they had met the wife of one of the Christmas tree guys. She was working behind the counter in a shop and when she learned where the Bennetts lived, she had gotten all excited. Her husband had been selling Christmas trees for 18 years just a few blocks from the Bennetts' apartment. The Bennetts didn't know him, though. They bought their tree at a different corner. Ellie's mom said she was going to invite the tree guys on their corner to dinner; she felt like she knew them that well!

This year, though, Hannah didn't want to help pick out the tree. She decided to help Mom unwrap the rest of the decorations. The box on top was labeled "Activity Scene." Hannah rolled her eyes. That's what she had called the nativity scene when she was little.

Hannah cleared off the spot on the table where they usually displayed it and pulled out the manger. As she placed the pieces in the barn, Hannah looked carefully at each face.

Even if the face on Mary's figurine did look more angelic than frightened, Mary must have been pretty scared. Hannah didn't think having a baby in a barn sounded so good. The stories gave the impression of nice, clean hay, but Hannah didn't think the hay could really be that clean. Just walking by the horses that gave carriage rides on the perimeter of Central Park was pretty smelly. And Hannah got to keep moving right past them. She didn't have to share a bed with them.

Every year at Christmastime, the priest gave a sermon on how Mary agreed to be Jesus' mom even when it would have been easier for her to say no. The point, Hannah knew, was that Mary should be a model for all humans—doing the right thing even when it would be easier not to. But, Hannah thought, God at least gave Mary an out. Mary could have said no, even if saying no wasn't what she should do.

God hadn't asked anybody if Mom could have cancer. Mom just got it. As far as Hannah was concerned, cancer stunk as badly as those horses in the stable. Hannah definitely would have told God "no", even if that was the easy way to go. No one should have to have a baby in a barn *or* get cancer.

Then she heard a lot of scratching on the front door.

"That must be the tree," Mom said, standing up to open the door.

The next thing Hannah heard was "umpf" as Dad brought the tree through the door and dropped the trunk on the floor.

Then, "Goodness, what a lot of branches! Come on in. I've got a place cleared for it right over here."

"Max," Dad said, giving Max a little push. "Keep walking. You've got to go on in so I can bring in the tree. Otherwise I'm going to trip and we're going to have branches everywhere! You can help once I get inside."

Hannah laughed when Max took one of the branches firmly by the hand and pranced with the Christmas tree to its place of honor in front of the windows.

"It's a pretty one, right, Hannah?" Max turned to her eagerly. "We took a lot of time picking, didn't we, Daddy?"

"Yes, indeed," Dad agreed. He put the stump end down on the floor, held the tree upright, shook out the branches. "We looked all of our options over very carefully before picking out just the right one."

Mom dug out the tree stand from one of the boxes and set it down. Dad carefully put the tree trunk between the screws and, while Max and Hannah held the tree straight on either side, tightened them.

Mom located the lights and Dad began stringing them. That was another argument Mom and Dad didn't have this year. Mom always wanted white lights, and Dad liked the colored ones. Dad usually won this battle, and he did again this year. Hannah didn't even see the box of white lights lying around anywhere. When she saw the bag of tinsel on top of one of the boxes, she knew Dad was going to get his way with that, too.

After a few adjustments to the light placement, they all stepped back to appreciate their handiwork.

"Now, we can't start decorating until we find the Christmas music." Mom said pointing to all the boxes. "The CDs are in there somewhere."

Max tore through all the tissue-wrapped items in one box, suddenly exclaiming, "Here they are, Mommy! I found them!" He took out a whole stack of compact discs and laid them proudly on the shelf below the stereo.

"I'll put them in," Hannah offered, dragging over a stool so she could reach the shelf where the stereo system was.

The stereo crooned *Dashing through the Snow* as the tree gradually gloried in its holiday finery.

Afterwards, as they admired their work, Mom announced that this occasion called for hot chocolate. "With lots of marshmallows, in honor of Jenny," she added, winking at Hannah.

Later that night, Hannah woke up and had to go to the bathroom. She noticed the tree lights were still on. Mom was standing in front of the tree in her pajamas, holding her glasses in her hands. Mom jumped when Hannah came over, "Oh, you startled me!" Mom said.

Mom noticed Hannah looking down at her hands. Mom was really blind without her glasses. A little embarrassed, Mom said. "I like to take off my glasses and look at the lights. It's the one time not being able to see is a good thing! The lights all blur and look like they're really twinkling." Then Mom smiled. "In my opinion, the white ones are more sparkly, but the colored ones don't leave much to complain about."

Mom put her arm around Hannah. "Your first Christmas, you were just a couple of months old. Anytime you got upset, we could just take you over to the tree, and you would stop crying. You were mesmerized by the lights."

"They're kind of like stars," Hannah whispered. "Like the stars we saw on our camping trip."

Mom nodded, and they stood there until the CD finished reminding them to *Have Yourself a Merry Little Christmas*.

The Friday of Mom's haircut came…and went. Even Max didn't remind her that they had missed the day. But he couldn't stand it on Saturday evening. "Mommy, when are we going to get to cut your hair? Now?" he asked hopefully.

"Ahhh, yes, the haircut. I was wondering when you'd remember." Mom patted the top of her head. She was curled up on the floor under a blanket, her head on a pillow, watching a Christmas special on TV with Max. "It seems such a shame to cut it when it's all still there."

"But, Mommy! You promised!" Max whined.

"Yes, I know."

Dad put down the paper he was reading on the sofa and looked down at Mom. "You know, Liz," he said, "you don't have to cut it. Who knows, maybe it won't fall out. Or, if it does start falling out, then the kids can cut it." Dad was always very practical.

"Daddy!" Max was alarmed at the direction of this discussion. "Mommy promised we could cut her hair."

"Max," Dad warned.

Max sulked in the chair, and Hannah could see his eyes were getting smaller and smaller.

"Oh, I know, I know." Mom stared up at the ceiling. "But we all know I'm going to lose my hair. Which is good. It means the drugs are killing the kind of cells they are supposed to, hopefully cancer cells as well as hair follicle cells. Besides, I really don't want to wake up one morning with a pile of hair on my pillow. I think that would make me really bummed, on top of wanting to throw up." Mom's first round of chemo had made her pretty sick.

Mom sighed. Then she rolled over and looked at Max. "Give me one more day with hair, OK? After dinner tomorrow night, we'll set up a hair salon, I promise. One more day."

Dad rubbed Mom's blanket with his toes.

"Mom," Hannah suddenly had an idea. "Mom, can I style your hair? You know, make it really pretty one more time before it's all gone?"

Mom nodded and made an effort to sit up while Hannah collected her hair styling equipment. But by the time Hannah had it all assembled, Mom was having a hard time holding up her head.

"Oh, Hannah," Mom said as she lay back down. "Sweetie, I just don't think I have the energy tonight for you to do this. I'm sorry. Tomorrow, though. Tomorrow I'll make sure I have enough energy to sit up for my fancy new 'do. I promise." Mom pulled the blanket up to her chin, and turned towards the TV.

127

When Hannah's eyes opened in the morning, she immediately saw the pile of hair accouterments Mom had waved off the night before. Hannah sighed and rolled over to face the wall. Hannah knew it was silly to feel abandoned, but Mom had practically ignored her the night before and just turned back to the TV. There wasn't even anything good on the television, just some stupid cartoon Christmas special she'd been watching with Max.

Hannah heard shuffling in the hall. Then the door flung open and Max ran in.

"Hannah! Hannah! Wake up! We gotta go to church!" Max announced.

Dad followed a minute later. He was buttoning the cuffs of his shirtsleeves. "Morning, Hannah-Banana," he said. "You ready to get up and go to church?"

Hannah rolled over again to face him. The brush, curling iron, and sparkly hair clips waited behind him lazily on the dresser. "Is Mom going with us?" she asked.

Dad shook his head. "No. Mom didn't have a good night last night, and she's finally gone to sleep. I don't want anyone to bother her."

Dad swooped Hannah up and out of her bunk. "Alright, Sleepyhead! Max and I let you sleep in, too, so we've all got to get a move on!" Dad placed Hannah down in the hallway by the bathroom, and she could hear Dad whistling as he went back to their bedroom to find something for Max to wear.

In a minute, Dad called to her, "Hannah! Hannah, can you come in here and help me pick something out for Max? I don't know what matches!"

Hannah couldn't pay attention in church, at least not to the priest. But she was extremely aware of all the hairstyles on every side of them. Hannah didn't know if Mom was going to feel like having her hair done today either, but if she did, Hannah wanted to be prepared.

Mrs. Olston's hair was always perfectly done, with a perky curl that bent the ends of her hair out right at the tops of her shoulders. Mrs. Schwein's hair was a mass of corkscrew curls. Hannah didn't think Mom's hair would do that, even if she used a curling iron on it. Mora, the teenager who occasionally babysat for them, had hair that fell in the most gorgeous chestnut sheet down her back. Hannah could almost see her reflection in it. Several of the women around them had short coifs. They were cute, Hannah thought, but Mom's hair was long-ish, so they didn't offer much in the way of possible style ideas.

Hannah saw several ponytails, and she noticed that some women had bangs. She kept squinting at people's faces. When she did, their faces blurred and it was easier for her to imagine their hairstyles with Mom's facial features. A few had clipped their hair up with elaborate hair jewels and barrettes. There were just so many options!

"Dad," Hannah asked on the way home, "how do you like Mom's hair best?"

"Uh," Dad looked surprised. "Mom's hair? How do I like it best? Well, let me think about that. What about you? How do you like it best?"

"That's what I'm trying to decide," Hannah explained. "I was looking at all the ladies at church trying to picture Mom wearing their hairdos. I just don't know how to style it for her."

Hannah's eyes opened wide and she raised her hands to emphasize the question. After she looked at Dad's face, Hannah added quickly, "If Mom wants it styled, that is."

"Max!" Dad called as his eyes darted up the sidewalk. "Max, that's far enough. Wait for us!"

Hannah watched as Max skidded to a stop in the middle of the sidewalk and posed like a statue. All the people approaching him had to make a point of going around his frozen form. When Hannah and Dad reached Max, Dad put a hand on Max's shoulder. "Hey, Buddy," Dad said, "you know you don't stop in the middle of the sidewalk. Where are you supposed to wait?"

Max pointed to the wall by a storefront, away from the crowds. "Then I'll be out of the way," Max explained.

Dad nodded in agreement. "Out of the way of people *and* cars," Dad emphasized.

As the three of them resumed walking, Hannah persisted with Dad. "So…how do you think I should do Mom's hair?"

"Well, Hannah, I just don't know if Mom's going to want to have her hair done. Her scalp is getting very tender, which means her hair is already beginning to fall out. I think the whole hair thing is very hard for Mom, and I don't want you to be disappointed."

Hannah thought a moment. "Well, if Mom does want her hair done, I'm going to curl it and then pull it back in a pretty barrette. That will be very elegant, and I think Mom should get to have elegant hair one more time."

When they entered their building, Charlie, the doorman said, "Hi, Bennetts! Liz just stepped out."

"You've seen Liz?" Dad asked in surprise.

"Yes, she just left." Charlie nodded. She said if I saw you to let you know she was going out for some ginger ale and Goldfish crackers. She said she'd be right back."

"Mom must be feeling better!" Hannah told Dad excitedly as they climbed the steps to their floor, "if she's gone out."

Dad nodded, "Maybe."

But Max shook his head. "I think Mommy is still sick. She always gives me ginger ale when my tummy doesn't feel good."

Dad nodded again. "Wonder why she didn't call us on my cell phone?" he said. "We could have picked up ginger ale on the way home." Dad pulled his cell phone out of his pocket. Then he rolled his eyes. "Oh."

"What?" Hannah asked.

"When I gave Max my cell phone to play with during church, I turned it off so he wouldn't accidentally make a call. I forgot to turn it back on. Even if Mom did call us, we wouldn't have gotten it."

As they were unlocking their door, Mom got off the elevator. "Hi, guys," she said a little weakly.

"Sorry, Liz," Dad said.

"Sorry for what?" Mom asked, approaching their door.

"Sorry I didn't get your call about picking up ginger ale."

"You couldn't have. I didn't call you. I thought about calling you, but then I decided that going for a short walk would be good for me. I knew the shop on the corner had both ginger ale and Goldfish, so I wouldn't have to go far."

"Does your tummy still hurt?" Max asked sympathetically, wrapping his arms around Mom's leg.

131

"Yes." Mom nodded. "It does. Ginger ale and, funnily enough, Goldfish crackers seem to help." Mom turned to Hannah, who was entering the apartment. "Are you OK, Sweetie?" Mom asked. "You seem awfully quiet."

"She's deciding what kind of hair you need," Max explained.

Mom's hand flew to her head. "Oh," she said.

Dad started, "But she knows…"

Hannah felt miniscule. It was obvious Mom didn't want her hair cut or styled. Even worse, Mom had forgotten all about it again. Hannah just wanted to curl up somewhere and be alone.

"What did you decide?" Mom asked, as they all entered the apartment and hung up their coats.

"You mean, what kind of hair style?" Hannah asked.

Mom nodded.

"Well, I was thinking about curling it and then pulling it back so it would look very elegant."

Dad looked dubious, but Mom put her hand on his arm. "I think that would be very pretty, Hannah. John," Mom added, turning to Dad and handing him her bag, "would you pour me a glass of this ginger ale and fix me a bowl of Goldfish, too?"

Max looked at the bag Mom had handed Dad with interest. Then he followed Dad into the kitchen. "Daddy, my tummy hurts a little, too. I think I need some ginger ale and Goldfish to make it feel better…"

132

ater that night after dinner, Mom was seated in the middle of the kitchen floor on a flattened-out plastic garbage bag. She ran her fingers through the curls Hannah had fixed for her earlier in the day. She smiled at Hannah. "I've felt so pretty all day, Sweetie. Thank you so much! Now, John, take my picture so we can remember what I look like with longer hair. It might be a while before I get these gorgeous locks back. Come on, Hannah and Max, I need a photo with my hair stylists!"

After the camera had flashed, Max jumped up. "Now can we cut your hair, Mommy? Can we? Right now?!"

Mom smiled. "Yes, but, remember, Max, you cut this side, and Hannah, you get this side. And, please be careful around my ears! I need my ears even if I don't need my hair!'

Dad put the camera down. He knelt down to Max's level. "Listen, Guys," Dad said to both of them, "I want you to be very careful with those scissors. You know that the chemotherapy means that Mom doesn't have as many white blood cells as normal, which means her body doesn't fight infections very easily. If you cut her skin, even accidentally, it could cause an infection that might be hard for her to shake. You have to be very careful. Absolutely no fooling around with the scissors, understand?"

Max and Hannah nodded solemnly, and then Mom interrupted, "John, pick up that camera. This is the only time these guys will ever be allowed to cut my hair, so you better record this milestone event!"

As Max immediately began sawing off Mom's curls with his scissors, Hannah stepped back. She wished now she had paid more attention to the short hairstyles she'd seen in church.

Mom smiled gently at her. "It's OK, Hannah, you can cut it. It won't hurt."

"Not even your scalp?" Hannah asked. "Dad said it might hurt your scalp."

"My scalp is tender," Mom said, "but it hurts all the time right now. Even when no one's messing with my hair, it hurts. Now cut away; I can't wait to see what style you're going to give me!"

Hannah made a few cuts, and then she stepped back again. Max was doing his best to give Mom a buzz cut with his scissors, but Hannah's side, for the most part, still hung to Mom's shoulder. Hannah realized she really didn't want to cut it. It had been fun styling Mom's hair, but cutting it seemed so permanent, almost cruel.

"You can cut my side, too, Max," Hannah offered.

"Really, Hannah?" Max asked excitedly as he moved his scissors into the still long side.

In a few minutes, Mom's hair was cut, all gone. Dad took the scissors away from Max and looked sadly at the pile of blonde hair on the plastic bag spread on the floor. Mom stood up and stretched. She rubbed her hand over her scalp. "Well, that took care of that, I guess. She looked at the hair on the plastic bag and sighed. "I had a lot of hair, didn't I?"

Hannah just looked at the jagged remains that topped Mom's head.

"I think I'll take a shower," Mom said starting towards the bathroom. "To get rid of the hair bits that are making my neck itch. I'll get the rest of it shaved tomorrow. Now I can start wearing all of my new hats!"

Hannah knew Mom was trying to sound cheerful, but it wasn't really working. In a minute the shower started going, and Hannah thought she heard a sob mixed in with the patter of water. Hannah slipped down the hall, crawled up on her bunk, and buried her head under her pillow. Nothing about cancer was turning out to be any fun.

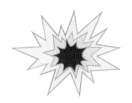

chapter 20
the beginnings of an
unusual friendship

after Christmas, things kind of settled into a routine, which, Hannah thought, was good. It was too bad that the routine was built around chemo, but it was good that there was a routine. All fall, none of them had known what was going to happen when. At least now they knew what to expect.

Thursdays were Mom's chemo day. Dad always took off work to go with her. Hannah and Max always had a play date on Thursday afternoons.

"Mommy, where are we going today?" Max asked one Thursday morning at breakfast.

"Today, Susan is going to pick you and Hannah up. You guys get to play with Ellie and Ken. I think she's asked Lucy and Ryan to come over too…"

"Pizza night!" Max cheered. Pizza night was an institution from the beginnings of their time in New York. Ellie and Ken, Lucy and Ryan, and Hannah and Max had all become friends about the same time, back when they all lived in the same building.

When they got together for dinner, pizza was usually on the menu because it was the only thing everyone would eat. Pizza night always meant a big mess and a lot of fun.

Not all of the Thursday morning directions were greeted with quite that much enthusiasm, though.

One Thursday, Mom answered, "Louise is going to pick you up. You too, Hannah. While Max and Ian play, you can play Battleship with Robert."

Max grinned delightedly, but Hannah stomped her foot. "Mom! I don't want to go home with a boy. I want to have a girl play date! Besides, I don't even like Battleship!"

"Well, you seemed to like it just fine when you and Will played it in the fall. I think you can give it another go."

"Mom! No! Please…can't I please go somewhere else? Please." Hannah didn't want any reminders of Will either.

"Hannah," Mom's voice sounded thin. "Hannah, I know. Believe it or not, I do understand. But, it was really nice of Louise to invite both of you over for dinner. Max and Ian are such good buddies, and you and Robert are the same age. Besides, it really is easier if you and Max are at the same place."

"Then let us go to Ellie's or Lucy's! Then I can have a girl play date and Max…"

"Hannah, you can't go to the same place every week. People have been so kind inviting both of you over every Thursday, and I don't want to wear out our welcome anywhere. Extra kids get tiring. Besides, they may have other plans today. People do have their own lives, you know."

On the way to Robert's house, Hannah kicked at a rock on the sidewalk. Max and Ian ran ahead and hid behind trashcans. When the stroller got close, they'd jump out in front of it to scare Betsy, Robert and Ian's little sister.

Hannah was concentrating so intensely on her rock that when something heavy pulled her down, she didn't know what it was.

"Hey! Oww..." Hannah cupped her hands protectively over her ripped tights and bleeding knees.

Louise looked at Robert in disbelief. "What were you doing? Look at Hannah's knees! Tell Hannah you're sorry!" Louise helped Hannah stand up and brushed off her tights. "We'll fix up your knees with some Band-Aids when we get home."

Hannah glared at Robert's back. Robert turned to his mom. "Sorry. I was trying to tag her so she'd race me to the corner."

"You need to tell Hannah you're sorry, not me." Louise informed him.

Then Robert looked over at Hannah. "Sorry," he said quickly. Then he added just as speedily, "If we beat those guys to the corner, we can scare them!"

"You didn't tag me! You pulled me down!" Hannah protested.

Louise said, "Hannah might not feel like running now that her knees are a mess."

"Do you?" Robert asked Hannah. Then he added quickly, "Feel like running?"

Hannah was still pretty mad and her knees did hurt. "No!" she snapped. "I can't and I don't."

Louise said, "Well, it's too late to run anyway. Our building's only a half of a block down."

When they all got upstairs, Max and Ian started playing trains, and Louise helped Hannah with her knees.

"Why don't you get out Battleship?" Louise suggested to Robert. "You and Hannah can try that. Hannah, do you know how to play?"

"I don't wanna play Battleship with a sissy ol' girl! Girls don't like to fight anyway!"

Hannah's eyes filled with tears. Her knees stung and she was being insulted. She didn't want to play that stupid Battleship either. Hannah wanted to go home.

Louise turned to Robert. "Look…" But before Louise could say anything else, there was a loud crash. They all ran to the back room.

Max and Ian had climbed up on the bookcase.

"What are you doing?" Louise asked, looking down at the huge pile of books and toys on the rug and then up at boys hanging from the shelves by one arm.

"We just wanted the special trains," Ian said. "But they're up there." He pointed to some boxes on the top shelves.

"There's a reason they're up there. So you can't get to them." Louise informed him. "You are lucky the bookcases are bolted to the wall! You could have been killed if they had fallen over. Ian, when you want something up high, what are you supposed to do?" Louise cleared a path from the doorway to the bookshelves.

"Ask you." Then Ian turned his head toward Max. "Max, if we climb up on the bunk bed and reach really high, we might…"

"You might fall off the top bunk and break your neck! Ian, the bed is on the other side of the room from the bookshelves. Even I can't reach them from there. You'd need a...a crane!" Louise finished.

Ian was still hanging off the bookshelf, holding on with one hand. He pretended his free hand was a crane, which sent him and Max into gales of laughter. Max laughed so hard he forgot to hold on and fell flat on his face on the floor.

"Ian, get down before you fall too. NOW!" Louise said as she hurried over to Max. He raised his head up from the floor.

"Are you OK?" she asked him.

"Owww," Max sniffled. "I need a boo-boo pack!" He sniffed again. "Do you have a boo-boo pack?"

Louise checked him for broken bones, and then said she'd get him an icepack because they didn't have a boo-boo pack.

"That's what a boo-boo pack is. It's an icepack! That's just what I need," Max said happily, his injury evidently healed.

When Louise went in the kitchen, they heard her exclaim, "Betsy! Oh, no! We were going to bake that for snack..."

Robert and Hannah ran from the back room to the kitchen. Betsy had opened the freezer door, which was close to the floor and climbed up the shelves inside to get to the refrigerator. Then she'd opened the refrigerator and climbed up those shelves, too. Now she was happily sitting on the counter, a bowl in her lap, scooping cookie dough into her mouth. She was covered in dough, and there was a generous sprinkling of chocolate chips all over the floor.

Robert picked up a few pieces of chocolate from the floor and wrinkled his nose. "Yum!"

The freezer shelves had tilted from Betsy's weight, and all the frozen food slid to the floor. Now it was covered in cookie dough that was escaping from the bowl. When Betsy had pulled the bowl from the fridge, she had knocked over a carton of eggs. Louise tried to turn it upright, but egg goo dripped on to the mess already on the floor.

"Ugh…" Robert said. "That's nasty. I don't think I want that for a snack."

Hannah silently agreed.

"Robert, can you guys go check on Max and Ian please? I have to get this cleaned up." Louise looked around wearily. Hannah guessed she was sorry she'd invited them for a play date after all.

When Hannah and Robert got to the bedroom again, Max was sitting on the floor looking up at Ian. "You better get down," Max warned Ian. "Your mommy's going to be mad."

Hannah and Robert saw why Max was so concerned. Ian had climbed up on the windowsill and was still trying to reach the trains. He looked like he was about to launch himself upwards from his new perch.

"Ian!" Robert shrieked. "You better get down NOW!"

Louise came running carrying a sticky Betsy on her hip. "What is it now?" she asked in exasperation.

When she saw Ian, she stood stock still, took a deep breath, and set the dough-covered Betsy down. She plucked Ian from the window and carried him into the living room. When she put him on the sofa, she said, "Don't move," in a voice no one would dare to cross.

Louise came back in the bedroom and picked Betsy up off the floor. Betsy hadn't moved because she was still busy pulling dough from her shirt and eating it. Robert and Hannah just looked at each other.

"I am taking Betsy into the kitchen and cleaning up the mess in there. Leave Ian alone on the sofa. I will deal with this," and she waved her hand at the mess in the room, "in a little while."

"Maybe we should pick up the toys," Hannah whispered to Robert after Louise left.

"Naww," he said. "She didn't say we had to."

"No, but…" Hannah started to stack some of the books.

Robert played with a train near where Max was sitting for a few minutes. Max just sat there, stunned into silence by the mess. It was a small blessing.

Then, without saying anything, Robert collected all the trains and put them in a basket. They made an assembly line. Hannah passed the books and loose toys to Max, and he handed them to Robert, who put them away on the shelf.

When they were done, Robert started to leave the room.

"I don't think we should go out there," Hannah said in a low voice.

"Why not?"

"Well, your mom said not to mess with Ian. And Ian's out there…" Hannah gestured towards the door.

"Yeah, but it's my apartment, too."

"Well…" Hannah was still pretty uncertain.

"Robert," Max asked from where he was still sitting on the floor. "Robert, will you teach me to play Battleship?"

Robert's eyes lit up. "Yeah!" he said excitedly. He got out the game and started to set up the pieces. But then his shoulders drooped. "We really need one more person, so you and I can be on the same team."

Hannah sighed deeply and rolled her eyes. She knew exactly where this was headed.

Max looked over at her. "Hannah, will you please play so I can be on Robert's team?" he asked in his sweetest voice.

Hannah sighed again and then nodded.

When Louise brought them home, Dad opened the door. "Come on in."

"Oh, I don't want to bother Liz," Louise said, blocking the door with her arms to keep Ian from running inside the apartment.

"Oh, Liz is a little tired, but it's not until later that she starts to feel bad. I know she wants to see you."

"OK, but guys, we're only staying a minute. Understand?" Louise gave Ian and Robert a fierce look.

As soon as Louise dropped her arms, Ian raced inside after Max.

Robert and Hannah stood in the living room while Louise gave Mom an edited version of the day's adventures. Robert even admitted in a whisper, "I think you beat me on that last race." He'd tagged Hannah on the way home, and this time, she'd given it all she had.

"Yeah, I know I did," Hannah said.

"You're not too bad, for a girl," Robert added.

"Thanks," Hannah replied. "You're OK, too."

"Are you going to come over and play *Battleship* again sometime?"

"If I have to." Hannah shrugged her shoulders.

"OK," Robert nodded.

They heard Max and Ian driving their trains down the hall. When they drove into the living room, Max looked up worriedly. "Mommy, why are you crying? Are you sad?"

Mom wiped her eyes. "No, Buddy, I'm laughing. Sometimes when you laugh really hard, you cry." Then she turned to Louise. "You are amazing! I hope your apartment survived." Mom shook her head, wiping her eyes. "Some days you just have to have the patience of a saint."

Seeing Mom laugh that hard made the whole play date worth it, Hannah thought. Even her injured knees.

Louise rounded up the boys to leave. Mom reminded Hannah and Max to say thank you. Robert tagged Ian and they sprinted off down the hall. Robert looked over his shoulder at Hannah and yelled, "I'll beat you next time!" As Dad shut the door, they saw Louise hurrying from behind with the stroller.

Mom waved Hannah over from the sofa. "So how was it? It sounds like quite an afternoon."

"It was all right," Hannah allowed.

Dad stepped out of the kitchen. "Dinner time!" he announced. "Hannah, will you please set the table? Max, do the napkins. Liz, do you want to sit with us?"

Mom shook her head. "I think I'll stay here on the sofa." From her position there, she could see into the dining area, so it was almost like they were all at dinner together.

"Daddy, what are we having?" Max asked. On chemo nights, someone almost always brought over dinner.

"Well," Dad said, "we are having lasagna, bread, salad, broccoli, and I believe we also have some dessert."

"What's the 'sert?" Max asked suspiciously. Sometimes the dessert was fruit, which, in Max's opinion, wasn't a proper way to end a meal.

"We will discover the identity of the dessert after we have consumed the more important parts of the meal," Dad informed him.

"But, 'sert is very important," Max told him. "I have to know what the 'sert is so I know if I have to try the other stuff." Mom and Dad didn't make them eat everything on their plates, but to get dessert, Hannah and Max did have to sample everything.

Mom laughed from the sofa. "I'm sure it'll be worth your effort, Buddy."

"Liz, you sure you don't want anything?" Dad asked Mom again, as the rest of them sat down to eat.

"No, I don't think so." Mom started to turn a bit green. Suddenly she got up and ran to the bathroom. Her reprieve from chemo's side effects was over and for the next few days, she would go into hibernation mode.

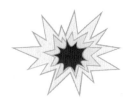

chapter 21
altered play dates

"Hannah, why can't we have a play date at your house?" Lydia asked a few days later at recess.

Hannah glanced up at Lydia. She knew Lydia was practically an only child since her older brother and sister didn't live at home any more. Hannah also knew that Lydia's mom didn't like her to have people over because their apartment was so small.

Lydia had been to Hannah's apartment once, back before the diagnosis. While the girls had eaten a snack, Lydia had talked nonstop to Mom, or really at Mom, until Mom finally shooed them away from the table. Lydia had been critical about everything in the apartment, from the books stacked on Mom and Dad's bedside tables to the art projects decorating the hall. Lydia's apartment must be extremely well organized, Hannah remembered thinking.

Hannah hadn't told Lydia or any of her other friends about the cancer. Some, like Ellie, Lucy, and Robert, knew because Mom had told their moms. Probably, Hannah was aware, a lot of kids knew, but none of those friends had mentioned it to her. Hannah didn't know why she didn't want

Lydia to know, but she knew she didn't. She did know Lydia wouldn't be at all discreet about it.

Mom had told Hannah's and Max's teachers immediately after the diagnosis. Mom said that if they ever wanted to stay in at lunch and talk to their teachers, they could. Hannah knew Mom had also told her teacher from the year before when Miss Lily showed up unannounced in her new class a few times just to say hi.

Hannah hated so many people knowing. She hated it when people asked her how Mom was doing. She hated it when people wanted to know how she, Hannah, was doing. It seemed like she couldn't do anything without cancer becoming front and center.

After her haircut, Mom had started wearing a baseball cap with some hair attached to the back of it. If you didn't know Mom was bald, you couldn't tell with her hat on. The hair was a lot blonder than her real hair, but no one seemed to notice. One kid in Hannah's class even mentioned that she liked Mom's new haircut. Hannah just smiled. That way she didn't have to tell a lie.

"We can have a play date at my house sometime." Hannah told Lydia. "We've just been awfully busy lately."

"Yeah, you've been awfully busy having play dates at a lot of other people's houses," Lydia retorted.

"I can't help it if a bunch of people want to have me over!"

"Like Robert? Yeah, Robert really wanted to have you over. And you really wanted to go, too, didn't you," Lydia said sarcastically.

"Hey, I like Robert. Not like *like*, you know, but I like him. He's funny. And besides he understands what it's like to have an annoying little brother."

That silenced Lydia for a minute because she didn't have a little brother, and Hannah thought that secretly Lydia would have liked to have one.

"Well, can I get on your busy social calendar then?" Lydia asked.

"I'll ask my mom," Hannah said slowly. "I don't know. We haven't really been having that many people over to our place recently."

"Why not?" Lydia was a little nosy and more than a bit bossy.

"Just because…because my mom's been busy." Hannah stammered.

Just then, Robert ran up and tagged Hannah. "You're it!' he yelled.

Taking advantage of a quick escape, Hannah took off after Robert full-speed ahead. He was so surprised that he didn't move fast enough, and Hannah caught him. "Ha! Got you back," Hannah squealed as she tagged him.

"Hannah's playing and I'm it!" Robert yelled at all the rest of the players, who scattered as he ran at them. He tagged Scottie, who immediately started chasing Hannah again. Hannah ran as hard as she could towards base, the equipment shed in the corner of the schoolyard. Out of the corner of her eye, she could see Lydia sitting on one of the benches watching.

Lydia claimed to like all the boys, but she really wasn't friends with any of them. Whenever she did join in the games most boys played at recess, Lydia always tried to change the rules. Hannah thought Lydia probably wanted to be playing tag right now. Should she wave Lydia over? If she did, Hannah knew that Lydia wouldn't just jump in and play; she'd want to change something in the game. Hannah was glad the whistle blew then for the end of recess. That meant she didn't have to make a tough decision.

As the class was climbing the stairs to the third floor, Lydia came up behind her in line. "You didn't even ask if you could play."

"Ask who if I could play? You?" Hannah was incredulous. "Robert tagged me. Basically he asked me!" Hannah retorted, annoyed by the accusation.

"Me. You didn't ask me," Lydia said in an annoyed tone. "That's not very polite. We were already talking and we were going to play together. Then you ran off and left me without even asking." Lydia said, folding her arms to her chest.

"We were talking, but we hadn't decided to play anything," Hannah protested. "Besides, Robert tagged me, I was it immediately. I couldn't ask you. Anyway, since when do I have to ask you who I can play with?"

"Well, I thought we were friends," Lydia said. "That's what friends do—play together. But now you don't want to play with me at recess and you won't invite me over. I guess we aren't really friends any more."

"Ladies, you'll notice we're back in the classroom. Those recess conversations need to wait until you're outside." Ms. Calde said.

149

Hannah's face flushed and she looked at her feet as she slid into her seat. She didn't ever get into trouble at school. Now Ms. Calde was scolding her on top of Lydia's fussing.

"Gees," Hannah thought, getting more and more irritated. "First Will, now Lydia. Pretty soon I'm not going to have anyone to talk to!"

Lydia elbowed Hannah as soon as Mom entered the playground at pick-up time. "Ask her now!" Lydia prompted.

"I'll ask her when we get home." Hannah said, waving to Ms. Calde and running over to Mom.

Lydia ran over too before Ms. Calde even noticed she'd left the group. "Go on. Ask her. Why not now?"

"Hi, Lydia," Mom said, giving Hannah a quick hug. "How are you?" Hannah looked at Mom—she was pretty pale. She wished Mom would wear some makeup and something besides her sweat pants. But Mom said her sweats were soft, and Hannah knew the chemo had made Mom's skin very tender.

Lydia elbowed Hannah again, and Mom raised her eyebrows at them. "What's up, girls?"

"Lydia wants to know if she can come over for a play date sometime soon," Hannah said, not really looking up at Mom. Hannah felt bad asking. Mom was so tired, especially late in the afternoons. And anyway, Hannah was pretty mad at Lydia. She didn't much want Lydia to come over.

"Hmmm," Mom said. "Let me look at my calendar and think about that. OK, girls? We'll find a time, but it might not be right away."

"Lydia!" Ms. Calde waved her back to the group, and Mom called for Max to come so they could head home.

On the way out of the schoolyard, Mom turned to Hannah. "You haven't had anyone to our place for a while. Would you like me to see if we can find a time between treatments for Lydia to come over?"

Hannah squirmed. She really didn't want Lydia to come. For one thing, Mom usually took off her baseball hat at home. If she wore it for too long, it gave her a headache. She usually wore a soft cap around the apartment because her head got so cold, and Mom had never liked being cold, even before cancer. With just the cap, though, Mom was bald and anyone looking at her could tell she was sick. Hannah had gotten used to it, but she knew Lydia would think Mom looked weird. And Mom without makeup and normal clothes would really tip Lydia off that something was up.

Besides, when something surprised Lydia, she often made mean comments. Hannah felt very protective of Mom. She didn't want Lydia to have the opportunity to say something rude about Mom's bald head.

a few weeks ago, they'd had a pizza night at Lucy's apartment. Max and Hannah had gone over for a play date in the afternoon, and then Mom had come over a little later. Mom was in the bedroom playing with the little kids, and she'd let Ryan see her head uncovered. Mom had even let Ryan touch it when he was curious about it.

Ryan had run out into the living room and announced excitedly, "Liz is letting us see her baldness! Come see!" before running back to the bedroom.

Lucy had wrinkled up her nose where the older kids were practicing their knitting and shook her head. "Uh-huh! *I'm* not going in there. I don't like baldies!"

Hannah thought that was a stupid thing to say. Lucy liked Mom fine before her hair fell out, and other than looking different, Mom was the same as she had been then. But Hannah wished Mom would keep her hat on, and Hannah had told her that on the way home that evening.

"Oh, Hannah, don't be silly. Of course I'll keep my hat on. It's just that Max and his friends think my head is funny. And it's good for them to see that I'm the same person with or without hair," Mom replied.

Privately, Hannah thought the same thing, but she didn't want anyone to make fun of Mom.

Mom shrugged. "It's just hair. I miss it a lot, but it's just hair."

"I like your shiny head!" Max had announced. "It looks like my head when I get a buzz cut!"

While they paused to wait for the light to turn green, at the corner, Max asked, "Mommy, can I get a buzz cut again so we can match?" Matching was very important to four-year-olds.

"You can get a buzz cut when the weather gets warmer. By then, my hair will have started growing again, so we really will match!"

Max was satisfied, and he raced ahead towards their building at the end of the block.

Hannah studied Mom's head with the baseball hat. "Mom, why don't you wear your wig?"

"Because it makes my head itch. The wig also doesn't work very well under hats, and with the cold weather, you know I really need a hat. It seems silly to wear a wig and a hat, and I'm definitely going to wear a hat. I guess I'm not much of a wig person." Mom had said.

Actually, Hannah was glad Mom didn't wear her wig. It didn't look like her at all. The baseball cap looked a lot more normal.

"Hannah?" Mom asked, bringing her back to the school-yard. "Do you want me to figure out a time to have Lydia over? Or someone else, maybe?"

"No. Not right now. Maybe later," Hannah told her. Lydia would definitely make fun of Mom, just like Lucy had. Mom might not care, but Hannah did.

Mom looked a little hurt, but she nodded.

Max started jumping up and down and pulling on her arm. "I want to have someone come over, too! Can I have someone over, Mommy? Can I?"

Mom patted his shoulders a little absently. "Yes, I'll figure something out." But she kept looking in Hannah's direction.

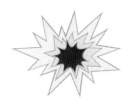

chapter 22
salmon pops

"**S**hould we get a movie?" Mom asked later that evening. She was stretched out on the couch rolling her neck around and stretching her arms.

Hannah looked up briefly from the book she was reading. "Ummm…" she muttered. Hannah always had a hard time transitioning from her books back to the real world.

Max, however, shrieked in delight, "Movie night?! We get to have movie night!" He started dancing around, shaking his arms like he had pompoms in them and cheering. "Yeah!"

"Hannah?" Mom asked, still under her blanket on the sofa, "What do you think?"

Hannah shook her head to clear out the story she was reading. "Sure. Yeah. But...," then she looked out the window at the branches on the trees iced with frost. "...I don't really want to go outside."

"Hannah!" Max protested, impatiently. "How can we get a movie if we don't go outside?"

Mom was still stretching her neck on the sofa. "Well, if you all know what you want, we could call the video store and have them deliver it. The only problem is that we don't have any dinner. I was thinking we could stop by the grocery store and you guys could pick out a frozen dinner for tonight."

"Like 'Dinners for Kids'?" Max asked in delight as he jumped up on to the coffee table. "We get 'Dinners for Kids' *and* movie night! Yeah!" He shook his pretend pompoms even more enthusiastically.

Frozen 'Dinners for Kids' was a treat mostly because they got to pick their own. People kept bringing meals over, so Mom hadn't had to cook in a long time. Mom was so tired that it was a good thing she didn't have to cook, Hannah thought, otherwise the Bennetts might not ever get a meal.

"But, Mom, what about Dad?" Hannah asked. Dad was not a fan of frozen meals because he claimed they just didn't fill him up.

"Remember? Dad's away tonight. He's fishing with Uncle Leland." Mom reminded Hannah.

"Mommy, when is Daddy coming back? I miss him. I wish he didn't have to go away!" Max said.

"He'll be back on Sunday, that's only two days away. Daddy hasn't had a break since all of this cancer stuff started. It's good for him to get away and go fishing for the weekend. Especially since I'm in between treatments right now."

"He should have taken me with him!" Max said. "Anyway, Mommy, how do you catch frozen fish? Frozen fish don't move."

"If he took you with him, it wouldn't be getting away, would it?" Mom laughed. Then she asked Max, "Frozen fish? Why do you think Daddy is going to be catching frozen fish?"

Max pointed out the window. "It's snowing, so the fish must be frozen!"

Hannah and Mom turned their heads towards the window in surprise. Hannah exclaimed, "It is snowing!"

"I didn't know it was supposed to snow today!" Mom said. Then she turned to Max. "The fish aren't frozen. The lake is frozen. Daddy and Leland will drill a hole in the ice and then drop their fishing lines into the hole. The fish are still moving under the ice."

"They must be pretty cold," Max observed.

"But it's not like they'll be fish popsicles!" Hannah laughed at Max.

Max pretended to hold a popsicle to his mouth. "Yummy, yummy fishy popsicle!" He twirled around licking at his imaginary popsicle.

"Salmon pops—now that's a product you won't find in a grocery store!" Hannah couldn't help but adding with a giggle.

Max slurped on his imaginary salmon pop some more.

Mom wrinkled up her nose. "Yuck! Now, is it going to be 'Dinners for Kids' and a movie for tonight? If so, I have to drag myself up off the sofa. If not...well, I guess we can have peanut butter sandwiches."

"Mom, can we have popcorn with our movie?" Hannah asked. She thought popcorn was the best part of movie night.

"No," Mom shook her head sleepily from the couch. "You have to have salmon pops tonight during the movie. Raw, frozen, salmon pops. Ummm...delicious! No popcorn, though. Absolutely not. Only salmon pops for this family."

"Daddy will like that!" Max said.

"Like raw salmon pops? Are you crazy? That's disgusting!" Hannah wrinkled up her nose.

"Yes, he will." Max argued. "He likes sushi and sushi is raw. Right, Mommy?"

"He likes sushi. I don't know if he would like raw salmon popsicles, but you never know. You can ask him when he gets back." Mom pried her eyes open again. "Ohhh, it's so hard to move…"

"Ok, Mommy," Max said, enthusiastically grabbing her hands, "I will help you! You have to get off the sofa so we can get our 'Dinners for Kids'!" He tugged at Mom's arms.

Mom smiled faintly and let Max pull her up to a sitting position. Then she shook her hands free from Max's grip. "M.D., would you please get my boots from the closet?" Mom let her head fall against the back of the sofa and closed her eyes.

"Here they are, Mommy!" Max announced.

Mom opened her eyes a crack. "Oh good. Thank you, Buddy. Now will you two get your boots and coats on?"

Mom lifted her foot to put on her boot. She looked like she was lifting a brick. This round of chemo had made her so tired that she spent most of the time on the couch. But by the time Max and Hannah had their winter gear on, Mom had gotten her boots on too and was standing up.

"Let's see, I just need my coat and my wallet. Where would my wallet be?"

Mom was usually very organized, but chemo had made her pretty scattered. She called it "chemo-brain." She didn't put things in the places she normally did, and then she could never remember where she had put them.

157

"Mommy!" Max said, "It's right here. Right on the bench where you usually put it."

"Well, that's unusual," Mom said. "Right where it's supposed to be, eh? Now what about my phone?"

Max dropped down to the floor to see if it had fallen under the bench, and Hannah went to check the spot by the plug where Mom charged it.

"No luck?" Mom asked. "Well, I guess I'll have to call it. Got your ears turned on?"

Max giggled. He loved this game—they listened for Mom's phone ringing and tried to track it down. One time, Max had found it in the freezer.

Hannah and Max traced the ringing into Mom's bedroom. Max picked up the phone and pushed the green button. "Hello? Mommy?" Max said into the receiver.

"Oh," Mom said, surprised. She wasn't expecting anyone to answer. She put the phone to her ear. "Hello?"

Max shook his head, giggling, "You put your phone on Daddy's dresser!"

"I did?" Mom shook her head. "I wonder why I did that. Oh, well. At least now we have it. We should go before I put something else some place weird."

Max grinned and turned the phone off.

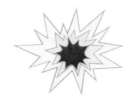

chapter 23
baldies

as they left their building, Max pointed to a bare-headed man on the corner. "Mommy, look! That man has cankser." Max nodded and looked very satisfied with himself for being so knowledgeable.

"Can*cer*," Hannah thought to herself, but didn't bother saying anything. She had given up hoping Max would ever learn how to say the word correctly.

"Oh, Max, honey. Don't point. That's not polite." Mom reached up to pull Max's hand down. "Besides, we have no idea whether or not that man has cancer. Why in the world would you think he does?" Mom continued as she took Max's hand to cross the street. The lights of the diner on the other side of the street cast a green glow on the falling snow.

"He's a baldy. Just like you. So of course he has cankser. That's why." Max said.

They stepped up on the curb right in front of the diner, and Mom turned sharply to face him. "Maximilian Douglas!" Mom snapped, using Max's full name, something she didn't do very often. "There are so many things wrong with that statement that I don't even know where to start!" The force of Mom's words made Hannah back up to the storefront.

Max looked surprised. Then his eyes narrowed and his lips trembled. The tears began to flow, freezing into tiny icicles on his cheeks. A family leaving the diner stared as they stepped around him. Max's shoulders heaved and in a split second, he was sobbing loudly.

It seemed like forever, but Mom finally started moving again as the anger drained from her face. She pulled Max into her arms, her puffy coat smothering him in a hug. "Oh, Buddy, I'm sorry." She tilted her head towards the diner. "What do you say we have dinner right here?"

Max was still crying. Suddenly Mom jerked her head up and her eyes darted down the street as they filled with panic. "Hannah? Hannah?" Mom called, her voice at least an octave higher than normal. But before Hannah could even move, Mom's eyes found her, still shivering against the wall. Suddenly, Mom's shoulders slumped and her eyes suddenly brimmed over with tears, too. Very tiredly, Mom wiped at the snow collecting on her glasses.

"Hannah, go on in. Ask them for a booth for three." Mom gestured at the diner door. Then she turned back to Max. "Come on, Max. Let's get some dinner. I'm sorry. I shouldn't have snapped. We can talk about it in the diner. We'll all feel better when we've eaten."

The waitress seated Hannah in a booth by the window. She could see the snowflake patterns sparkling in the streetlights. She could also see Mom and Max still standing as the snow fell. Mom had her arm around Max, but Max was stiff.

"Come on, Max," Hannah thought. "Just come on in." But she knew how he felt. She wasn't sure why Mom had snapped at Max. Getting snapped at was painful, especially if they didn't know what they'd done wrong.

Hannah pressed her face to the window and flattened her nose. Mom saw her and smiled gratefully. Mom said something and pointed to Hannah's face through the glass. Max looked up, and Hannah stuck out her tongue, leaving a big, wet, slurpy spot on the window. Mom grimaced and Max giggled. He wiped his nose with the back of his mitten—Hannah saw Mom grimace again but she didn't say anything. They stepped toward the door of the restaurant.

Max's eyes filled again when the waitress handed him a menu. "But, I really wanted 'Dinners for Kids,'" he sniffled.

Mom reached over and ruffled his hair. "Tomorrow night we can have 'Dinners for Kids.' Daddy will still be fishing tomorrow, and we'll go to the grocery in the morning and have them for dinnertime."

Max wiped his eyes with the back of his hand and nodded.

Once they had all placed their orders, Mom said, "Max, I'm really sorry. I overreacted. That wasn't very nice of me. But…"

"No buts, Mom," Hannah interrupted, mimicking Mom. "Just say you're sorry and that's that." Whenever Max or Hannah had to apologize for something, Mom would never let them add a *but* to tell why they had done it. Mom said when you're really sorry, you're sorry and you shouldn't be worried about where the blame goes.

Mom's mouth closed tight right in the middle of her next word, and she looked away from the table.

"Mommy, are you really sorry?" Max asked. "Because if you're really sorry, then you shouldn't try to blame me for you getting mad."

Mom took a deep breath and looked back at them. "Yes, I am really sorry. I snapped, and I shouldn't have. I should have told you politely why I was upset." She looked right at Max. "Will you forgive me?"

Max nodded happily. "I love you, Mommy."

"I love you too, Max, but we do have to talk about what you said."

Max took a big slurp of milk through his straw. "Hey," Hannah turned to him. "No slurping. That's gross."

"But I like to slurp," Max giggled.

"Ok, Guys," Mom said, her voice wearing a little thin, "we aren't talking about slurping here."

Just then the waitress brought out the burgers and fries. She put a plate of plain pasta in front of Mom. Mom's stomach was pretty tender from the chemo. But the grilled burgers made Hannah's nose sing, and right at that moment, Hannah thought the diner dinner even beat "Dinners for Kids."

As Hannah picked up her burger, she saw Mom close her eyes and wrinkle up her nose. Mom covered her mouth and scrambled over Max to get out of the booth. She stuttered over her shoulder, "I'll…" and ran for the bathroom.

"I don't think Mom feels very good," Hannah said to Max, who was dumping catsup on his fries.

When Mom returned, she took a huge swallow of her ginger ale and asked the waitress to wrap up their food and bring them a check.

"But, Mommy, I'm really hungry," Max whined, and his eyes shrank.

"Don't cry again, Max," Hannah whispered. "Just put your coat on."

"You can eat dinner at home," Mom said, ushering them out of the restaurant. "The smells in here are making me nauseous."

Later that night, Mom had resumed what Dad called her "chemo position." She was stretched out on the couch, covered with a blanket, with the telephone, TV remote, a book, and something to drink, all within easy reach. Max and Hannah were settled in next to her as the movie (which they had delivered) finished.

M.D. took the disc out of the DVD player. "Mom," Hannah said, inspecting the popcorn bowl for any remaining kernels, "what was wrong with what Max said tonight? I didn't think he said anything bad."

Max shook his head vigorously. "I didn't say anything bad. It wasn't bad at all. That man was a baldy. He didn't have any hair."

Mom said, "Well, even if he didn't have hair, it's not very nice to call him a 'baldy,' is it? I don't really want people to call me a baldy. And there are plenty of people who are bald who don't have cancer."

"Like who?" Max wanted to know.

"Think of Uncle Pete, and… what about Mr. Jack who lives down the hall?"

Max shook his head. "Uncle Pete's not really bald. He has fringe all the way around. And Mr. Jack is only bald on the very top. He has regular hair everywhere else. Besides he puts his other hair on top of the bald spot." Max tried to flip his own hair over his scalp, demonstrating Mr. Jack's comb-over.

Hannah saw Mom hide a smile. "The point is," Mom started again, "that being bald doesn't mean you have cancer. And, plenty of people have cancer who aren't bald."

Max said, "Well, you have cansker, and you're bald."

"But I wasn't bald when I first learned I had cancer, and I most certainly had hair before that when we didn't even know the cancer was in my body. Besides, some people get their cancer treated with medicines that don't make you lose your hair."

"So," Hannah interrupted, "you just don't want Max to call anyone a baldy?"

"I definitely don't want him to call anyone a baldy," Mom said. "I don't like that word. It just doesn't sound nice. But it's more than that. Everybody is different in some way. For me, right now, it's being bald. And I don't like it when people point out that difference. It's kind of like staring or pointing. It's rude."

"But, Mom, I'm tall. I don't care if people say something about me being tall," Hannah protested. She didn't want to tell Mom that Lucy had called her a baldy.

Mom paused in her lecture and then nodded slightly, thinking. "Yeah, you're right—that's a difference that doesn't seem to matter. But there are some differences it's not nice to draw attention to—like being heavy, or having a bad scar, or being bald. For some reason, people often think that those type of characteristics, which are really just on the surface, mean there's something different about the person on the inside."

Mom studied the ceiling and thought a minute. "I guess the reason I got so upset earlier was because Max jumped to a conclusion about that man when he didn't have any real information to make that statement. I don't want you guys to judge people before you know them. Calling him a baldy gave him a label, and labels aren't very nice, especially since we don't even know the man. And it just happens to be a label I am very sensitive to right now."

There was something familiar about what Mom was talking about but Hannah couldn't quite place her finger on it. She did think Mom had gotten worked up over nothing. Not only did that man not know Max was labeling him, he probably wouldn't have even cared. The guy was bald. Frankly, Hannah thought the guy was flaunting it since he wasn't wearing a hat in the snow.

Hannah didn't really like the word "baldy" either and certainly not when someone called Mom one. But it wasn't a bad word or anything. She didn't think it was worth all this fuss.

"Look," Mom said, "I told you I overreacted and I'm sorry. I guess I'm just sensitive about hair right now—even though I know it's just hair and I know it will grow back." Mom pulled off her cap and rubbed her shiny scalp. "Just be careful judging people based on their looks. That's never a good idea."

Mom closed her eyes for a minute and then shook her head, adding, "I just don't understand why that guy wasn't wearing a hat. In that snow, even if I had hair, my head would have been an ice cube!" Mom shivered dramatically and pulled the blanket up to her chin.

Hannah and Max both reached over and stroked her smooth skull. "I like you being a baldy," Max said. "Now your head is slippery!"

"She's not a baldy!" Hannah said, punching him on the arm. "She may be bald, but she's not a baldy!"

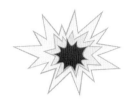

chapter 24
the great reveal

a few days later, Scottie and Hannah were sitting at the table listening to Lydia drone on. Hannah glanced out the window longingly. Snow was piled up on the playground equipment, which explained why they were stuck indoors for recess.

"We're starting a new club," Lydia babbled. "I'm the president. You two can be in it, and then we'll have to vote on the other members. I'll have two votes and each of you can have one."

Suddenly Scottie jumped up. "That's not fair!" He banged his fist on the table. "Why should you get more votes? Besides why would we even want to be in your stupid club?"

Lydia straightened up her shoulders and flipped her long hair behind her shoulders. "Well, you don't have to be in my club if you don't want to," she snapped. There are lots of people who will want to be in it. You'll see...and for that matter, we might not even vote you in!" Lydia's chair fell over when she stood up and stormed off.

Scottie looked at Hannah and sighed. "Sometimes she's just too big for her britches." Hannah giggled at the thought of Lydia trying to squirm into her pants.

Scottie narrowed his eyes and looked harder at Hannah. "Hey!" he said in surprise, "you're laughing. You don't do that much any more."

"My mom has cancer." It just slipped out.

Scottie's mouth opened in a silent, surprised "O."

"That's why Mom has the haircut, because it's fake. She actually doesn't have any hair. The hair is attached to the hat."

Scottie nodded slowly, his mouth still wide open.

"That's also why I haven't been having any play dates at my house. Mom's too tired. The chemo makes her white blood cell count lower. That means she could get sick more easily if she's exposed to germs."

Hannah raised her eyes from the table and looked at Scottie. "You can close your mouth, you know," she reminded him.

Scottie snapped his lips shut. Then he asked, "What is 'white blood cell count'?"

"Remember from science? White blood cells make up the part of your blood that fights infections. Chemo affects those cells along with cancer cells, so right now it's a lot easier for Mom to get sick." Hannah answered.

"Why would chemo hurt something that is supposed to keep you well?"

Hannah sighed. "Chemo actually prevents white blood cells from maturing," Hannah recited, feeling a little like a cancer encyclopedia. "It also kills all fast-growing cells because cancer cells grow fast. That's why you lose your hair."

Scottie looked puzzled.

"Hair cells multiply quickly, just like cancer cells," Hannah continued her recitation. "So chemo does them in. But it doesn't kill white blood cells, it just keeps them from getting mature enough to fight infection effectively."

"But your mom picks you up from school," Scottie protested. "And drops you off," he added. "That seems pretty normal."

"Yeah. Mom wants us to be as normal as possible. So when she's feeling OK, she picks us up but doesn't really hang around. That way she's not exposed to as many germs. But nothing's normal right now, that's for sure."

"Does Lydia know?" Scottie asked, after a minute.

"I haven't told her," Hannah replied.

Scottie nodded again. "She'd never let you forget it."

"I know. Sometimes it feels like cancer is my whole life right now. And I don't want to be reminded of it when I don't have to be."

"But if she knew, it might shut her up about the play dates," Scottie said thoughtfully.

"Maybe. But you know Lydia. She likes to be the one in charge. If I told her, she would probably try to figure out some way to take control." Hannah sighed again.

"Why don't you get your mom's doctor's number for her? Then she can call him and have a personal consultation," Scottie smirked.

Hannah giggled again. Scottie smiled broadly and thumped the table with his fist. "Lydia's advice column. Now that's what she should do!" He continued enthusiastically, "Lydia should publish her proclamations so that all of New York City can take advantage of her great wisdom!"

They were both bent over laughing when Lydia stalked back to the table. "What are you two snorting about?" she asked through her teeth.

"My mom has cancer," Hannah told Lydia through her giggles.

Lydia looked shocked. Scottie righted the overturned chair just as Lydia sat down hard. "What?"

"My mom has cancer," Hannah repeated. The giggles vanished, and she said somberly, "That's why you can't come over for a play date right now."

"But... people who have cancer are bald," Lydia protested.

"Mom *is* bald. The hair is attached to her hat. It's fake." Hannah added, "And, anyway, not all people who have cancer are bald. Not all chemotherapy drugs make you bald."

"But, but..." Hannah could see Lydia struggling with this new information. Lydia was in the uncomfortable position of not being on top of the situation for a change. "But people who have cancer are sick. Your mom picks you up. People who have cancer are dying!" Lydia looked right at Hannah, as if Lydia was the one imparting new information.

"Lydia!" Scottie fumed.

"She's not dying." Hannah interrupted calmly. "Cancer is really bad, and it can make you die. But Mom's not dying. She's getting chemotherapy to make sure the doctors got all the cancer when they did the surgery. Any cancer cells that are left will hopefully get zapped by the chemo. Some days Mom feels ok, and some days she feels lousy. But it's the chemo that does that, not the cancer. Mom's going to be fine."

Lydia looked up at Hannah. "Wow," Lydia whispered.

Scottie winked at Hannah. Hannah had finally achieved the impossible—Lydia was almost speechless.

Hannah was happy that the whistle blew for the end of recess so she didn't have to try to figure out how to change the subject.

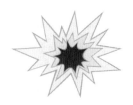

chapter 25
stereotypes

ater that night, Hannah was lying on the living room floor looking up at the ceiling. Dad was putting Max to bed, so it was blessedly quiet for a change. Hannah thought about Lydia and what she had said about Mom dying. Hannah wondered why she hadn't gotten mad at Lydia, but when Will had said it, Hannah had been furious. She felt bad that she had gotten so mad at Will.

That uncomfortable feeling that she was missing something nagged at her again. It was as if she could see an important piece of a puzzle in the distance but it was still blurry. Hannah shook her head slightly, trying to clear her mind, but she couldn't shake off that nagging feeling. Somehow, something just wasn't quite clear yet.

Hannah went back to thinking about Will and Lydia. Hannah had been overly sensitive about Mom's dying with Will, just like when Mom had snapped at Max the other night. Mom had been overly sensitive about being bald with Max. Hannah laughed at herself. You couldn't really compare being bald and death, but somehow both of them were all mixed up with cancer.

"Mom," Hannah asked suddenly, "are we going to see Will again soon?"

Mom was doing her arm stretches against the wall. "Umm…" she muttered between reaches. "At some point. We don't have any plans with them right now." Mom grasped her hands together over her head, pulled, and counted to ten. Then she sat down on the sofa. "Why? You haven't even mentioned him since Thanksgiving. I thought you two had a falling out of some sort."

"I think I overreacted to something he said. Maybe I need to apologize."

"Ahh," Mom grinned. "The old overreaction requiring an apology. I don't know anyone else who has ever had to do that!" Mom tapped her own chest with her index finger ruefully and then rubbed the top of Hannah's head with her foot. "You could call or write him a letter…" Mom suggested. Hannah screwed up her mouth. "Or email him," Mom added.

"Mom, what's the worst part of cancer for you, being bald or…?"

"Or what?" Mom prompted after a minute.

"Well, or…" Hannah wondered how could she ask her mom if she was afraid of dying.

Mom stretched out on the floor beside Hannah. "Or being afraid of dying?" Mom supplied.

Hannah sat up in surprise. "How did you know I was thinking that?!"

"Because I think about it. And you're a thinker, too. So it stands to reason that you would think about it as well."

Hannah lay back down on the floor and rested her head on Mom's shoulder. "Well…" she prompted Mom.

"You know," Mom laughed, "the hardest part is probably being bald. I guess because then everyone knows you do have cancer. And my head is always cold!"

"But you do think about dying?" Hannah persisted.

"Of course. Lots of people lose the cancer fight. There's no question about that. And I don't want to leave you and Max and Dad any time soon. I want to see you grow up and have your own children, and I want to be able to travel the whole world with Dad and live in lots of interesting places."

Mom continued, "I get scared that maybe the doctors missed a cancer cell that's going to start growing somewhere that's particularly hard to treat. I also worry that something I did caused the cancer. I want to know what that was so I can stop doing it and so I can keep you guys from doing it."

Mom paused a moment and then continued thoughtfully, "I'm not really afraid of dying. I believe that Heaven will be better than Earth, and I believe that we will finally understand so much that we don't understand now."

Mom paused again and then added, "But I'm not ready to die, not by a long shot. I sure hope my time on Earth isn't over. Besides having more time with you guys, I hope I can do something to help humanity. I hope that's in the plan, too!"

"Being bald is harder than all that?" Hannah asked, incredulously.

"Yeah," Mom laughed, arching her neck back and rolling her head to the side to look at Hannah. "It is. Because I don't think about that stuff all the time, but every time I reach up to run my fingers through my hair, or I look in the mirror, or I get ready to go somewhere, I think about being bald. And I know that when other people see that I'm bald, they know I have cancer and probably think I'm dying. That's what used to go through my head whenever I saw a bald woman. I want people to know I am not dying. Even more importantly, I really don't want people to feel sorry for me!"

Mom took a deep breath. When she let it out, she grinned at Hannah, "Besides, being bald means my head is..."

"I know, I know," Hannah nodded, "your head is perpetually cold."

Then Hannah squinted past Mom's face. That feeling pushed relentlessly inside her head. Suddenly Hannah sat straight up. "Stereotypes!" Hannah exclaimed excitedly, looking up at Mom.

Mom waited for Hannah to explain.

"That's what Max did to that man the other night. Max stereotyped him because Max decided the man had cancer just because he was bald. You don't like being stereotyped. You don't want people to think you are dying just because you are bald."

Hannah lay back down on the floor, feeling as though she had solved a great mystery.

Mom squeezed Hannah's shoulders gently. "I hadn't thought about it like that. But, yes. I guess the word 'baldy' implies cancer to me, and cancer in turn implies dying."

Mom added thoughtfully, "Even though chemo is coming to an end in a few weeks, it isn't going to feel like cancer's really over until I get my hair back."

"Because then people won't know!" Hannah sat up excitedly again.

"Won't know what?"

"When you have hair again, people won't know that you've had cancer. At least they won't know just by looking at you," Hannah said slowly. "Then they won't be able to stereotype you as a cancer..."

"Victim," Mom whispered softly.

Hannah looked down at her, surprised. Mom smiled ruefully. "Sometimes that's what I feel like—a victim—of this random disease." Mom stopped talking for a moment and then nodded reflectively. "You know, you're absolutely right. Cancer won't feel like it's over until my hair comes back. With a full head of hair, I won't be stereotyped as a cancer patient."

"Ms. Calde says the only way to break stereotypes is to get to know the people you are stereotyping," Hannah mused.

She thought some more. "You know, I don't think it's the actual words that are so bad." Hannah stretched her neck to the side, trying to grasp another important thought that was trying to push its way out.

"It's what people think a stereotype means that is bad. You think the word 'baldy' means people think you are dying. That's not what Max thought the other night. He just thought that guy had cancer."

"And," Mom agreed, "Max doesn't necessarily think there's a connection between cancer and death."

Hannah sat up again, excitedly. "It's like me. I'm tall, but because being tall doesn't mean anything bad to me, it doesn't matter if someone calls me *tall*."

Mom nodded, thinking over Hannah's revelation. "I think you're on to an important idea."

Hannah turned to Mom and asked hopefully, "Will everything be normal when your hair grows back?"

"Oh, Sweetie, I don't think everything will ever feel exactly the same again. But we'll make a new kind of normal, and some of it will be even better than it was before."

"Will the new normal also be finding a way to help..." Hannah's voice trailed off, because she wasn't quite sure what Mom had meant.

"Help humanity?" Mom finished for her. "Yes, I hope so. Maybe that can be something we figure out together— how we can use our good fortune to make life better for someone else."

Mom smiled at Hannah, who was still arching her neck backwards and then rolling her shoulders. "That's a tall order, and Dad would probably say I sound awfully idealistic," Mom said. "But think how much people have helped us. Not only our friends, with all the meals and play dates, prayers, and support, but also all the scientists who've figured out how to treat cancer as effectively as they have. Even the people who thought up the idea of the baseball cap with the hair—now that's been a true godsend. Every little thing becomes so important."

Mom shook away her own thoughts and stood up. She reached for Hannah's hands and pulled her to a standing position. "Ok, Missy, come on. It's bedtime. You can send that email to Will tomorrow."

aybe," Hannah said to herself as she crawled under the comforter, "maybe that's why I got so mad at Will at Thanksgiving when he said Mom was dying. I didn't know it, but back then I believed that all people who have cancer do die. When he said what he said, I got scared."

177

"But now," Hannah thought, closely observing the street lights filter through the branches dancing in their shadowy ballet, "now, I know Mom, and I know some of her email friends, and they aren't all dying. Sure," Hannah reminded herself, "some of them are pretty sick. But not all of them. Lots of them have been survivors for years."

Hannah listened to the traffic symphony outside the window for a while. "That must be why I didn't get mad at Lydia today. Because now I know more about cancer. I know Mom isn't dying, at least not right now. Ms. Calde would say I'm breaking a stereotype."

Hannah grinned for a moment and then whispered to herself as she drifted off. "All stereotypes ought to be broken. No, not just broken, but smashed, smashed into a million little pieces! Particularly when they involve your mom…"

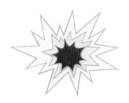

chapter 26
spring beginnings

"Hannah, look!" Max poked her early one Saturday morning.

Hannah was on the fringes of sleep, but as Max leaned over from the top of the bunk bed ladder to open the blinds, the bright sunshine forced her eyes open.

"Hannah! Look!" Max repeated urgently tapping on the window.

"What is it? What time is it?" Hannah murmured sleepily from under the covers.

"Look at the tree!"

"What tree?"

"This tree, the one right here." Max stopped his tapping and pointed out the window.

Hannah propped herself up on her elbow and let her eyes adjust to the light. "Yeah, I see the tree. The same tree that's always there. What about it?" she asked impatiently.

Then Hannah squinted at the clock. "Oh Max! It's not even 8:00 a.m.! On a Saturday! You know I like to sleep in on Saturdays—it's the only morning I can!"

"But Hannah, look, the tree is starting to be green. See, right there." Max pointed outside.

Hannah peered through the blinds a little more closely. Faint green buds were beginning to appear on the long, gray arms of the branches.

"Hannah, green trees mean it's spring! We're getting to spring! Yeah!" Max danced around the room singing at the top of his lungs, "Spring, spring, spring! I love spring!" Then he stopped in the middle of the floor and gazed up at the top bunk. "Do you think Mommy will let me wear shorts today?" Then he added hopefully, "It *is* spring."

"It's not spring yet," Hannah sighed. "The tree is starting to bud, but it's still cold outside, and anyway, spring doesn't start until the Spring Equinox."

"What's that?" Max demanded.

"When the days start getting longer," Hannah said, her voice muffled by the covers.

"Longer?" Max puzzled. He pulled a measuring tape from the toy basket. "How much longer?" he asked pushing the tape towards Hannah's head.

"Not that kind of longer, Silly," Hannah said. "Longer, as in more daylight. It's on the calendar."

As Hannah started to burrow into her covers again, Max demanded, "Show me!" and marched into the kitchen to look at the calendar on the refrigerator.

Hannah reluctantly followed, knowing her traditional Saturday morning lie-in wasn't going to happen. As she found March 20th, she realized they were just a few days away from the start of spring. Hannah lifted the calendar page and saw that Mom's last chemo was just a few weeks away. She picked up a yellow crayon and circled April 17th.

"We should have a party," she suggested to no one in particular. "An end-of-chemo party."

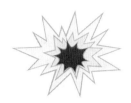

chapter 27
revolutionary stereotypes

"**m**s. Calde wants us to see the people behind the stereotype, right? So, first we have to figure out what the stereotype is. What's the stereotype of the Patriots?" Hannah asked her group impatiently. There weren't too many more History Project group meetings before show time.

Sam looked worriedly at Hannah. He didn't like how what she was saying might change their outline. Scottie stared hard at her, waiting for more information, and Mary chewed on her lip thoughtfully.

"When you think of the Patriots, what's the first thing you think of?" Hannah urged.

"A football team. A very cocky football team." Scottie grimaced under his breath. He was a hardcore New York Giants fan.

Hannah made a face at him. Of all the kids in their group, she was counting on his support.

Scottie swallowed his grin. "Farmers," he supplied instead. "The Patriots were very poor farmers."

"George Washington wasn't poor!" Sam protested. "He was rich, or at least his wife was," Sam corrected himself.

"I know that," Scottie replied, a little annoyed. "But Hannah asked for the first thing I thought. The first thing I thought was a poor farmer. And anyway, George Washington *was* a farmer."

"A plantation owner with slaves is a bit different from a poor farmer," Sam pointed out.

"I didn't say George Washington was a poor farmer, just that he was a farmer," Scottie argued.

Hannah jumped in. "That's it! Not all of the Patriots were poor or farmers." She paused and looked at Sam pointedly, "Or poor farmers. I think in our presentation we should talk about some Patriots who weren't poor and who weren't farmers."

Mary interrupted, "What about the Redcoats? Some of them were just over here doing what they were supposed to do and then this war started. I don't think all of them were as mean as the books say."

Scottie turned to face Mary. "I hadn't thought about the people on the other side. I guess that's another stereotype," he mused.

Even Sam was beginning to nod. "You know," he said slowly, "if the British had really wanted to keep the Colonies, they could have sent over a lot more soldiers and pretty much squashed the Patriots flat. So, yeah, the Patriots won, but the British didn't exactly put their whole heart into it."

"Maybe," Mary said, "we should start our presentation with some of the stereotypes most kids probably think, and then show how they weren't true."

"And," Hannah added suddenly, "why they were kind of true."

The group turned to her, confused. "But stereotypes aren't true," Mary protested.

"I think that some part of the stereotype has to be true at least some of the time, otherwise it wouldn't get to be a stereotype," Hannah said. "It might just be a little piece. Like some Patriots were poor farmers and some of the Redcoats were probably mean."

In her head, she thought, "Like some people with cancer do die."

"Or," Mary chewed on her lip some more. "Sometimes, the other side makes the stereotype."

Hannah, Scottie, and Sam looked at Mary questioningly.

"Well, the Patriots didn't want anyone to like the Redcoats, so maybe they spread the idea that all of the Redcoats were mean."

Sam nodded. "And the Redcoats didn't want anyone else to join the Patriots' side, so they probably told everyone that the Patriots were a rag-tag army of poor farmers and there was no way they could win the war."

After a minute, Scottie agreed. "You have to see both sides to figure out the truth. We should show both sides and let people make their own decisions. Now, how are we going to divide this up?"

Hannah sighed. "I still haven't gotten to Thomas Paine Park, but I have done some research on the guy. He wasn't a farmer; he was a writer. But he was poor." She looked down at her notes. "He wrote *Common Sense*, a pamphlet that was really important in getting many of the people living in the colonies to support the War for Independence."

"So," Mary said, "let's start with him, since he seems to have been such an important part of getting everything started. We can show how he…"

"Busts a bunch of the stereotypes!" Scottie interrupted. "You know, he was a writer, not a farmer. And if his article was so important in getting the Revolution started, obviously, the Patriots weren't all dumb farmers who couldn't read! They had to read it to know what it said."

Even Sam was nodding. He reassessed the outline. "Look, guys. This is how I think our presentation should go…"

The Revolutionary War group bent their heads over Sam's desk and started to make real progress on their project.

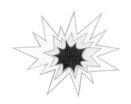

chapter 28
triskaidekaphobia

dad rummaged through his pockets looking for his MetroCard, as he, Hannah, and Max descended into underground New York. Hannah clutched her own card tight in her palm.

"I want my own MetroCard!" Max announced, dangling off the stair rail.

"Keep moving, Buddy," Dad warned. "There are people behind you."

"But, Daddy…"

"You're too little for your own MetroCard!" Hannah snapped, grabbing Max's hand. She was annoyed that Max had to come. After all, it was *her* history project. Mom was taking a nap, but surely Max could have stayed home while Mom slept.

"No, I'm…" Fortunately, Max was diverted by sounds drifting up from the subway platform. "I want to see the music!" Max dropped Hannah's hand and ducked under the turnstile.

"Max, wait!" Dad called, swiping his own card. He rushed through the rotating metal bars and glanced back at

Hannah. Her card wouldn't swipe properly, and the bars held fast, preventing her from crossing to the platform.

Hannah blinked rapidly, holding back tears of frustration, while she ran her card through another time.

Suddenly a worn hand rested gently on her shoulder.

"Here, Honey," the stranger said, "Give it just a minute before you swipe it again. Sometimes these machines just need a little rest."

After a moment, the man said, "Now try it. That's right, nice and slow. There you go." He pointed towards Dad, who was coming towards her with Max in tow. "Your dad's right there, and that little escape artist must be your brother." With a deep laugh, the man nudged her through the turnstile.

On the other side, Hannah turned to thank the man, but no one was there. All she saw was a pair of baggy khaki trousers and fraying sandals melting into the crowd.

Dad ran up to her, gripping Max's hand. "Hannah! Are you OK?" Before she could answer, Dad turned to Max, "Don't you ever run ahead like that again, Young Man! You could fall onto the tracks. You could get lost—it can be dangerous down here!"

"Hannah!" Max exclaimed, ignoring Dad. "They're playing *Feelin' Groovy*! You know, the song about the bridge that's kind of near our building!" After a pause, Max asked, "Which bridge is it that's near our building?"

"The 59th Street Bridge," Hannah replied shortly.

Then Max faced Dad and implored, "Daddy, can we put some money in their guitar case? Please?"

As Hannah slid her MetroCard back into her pocket, some coins jingled deep in the folds of the fabric. She retrieved two quarters and three dimes and glanced back to the turnstile, where she'd just been rescued. "Here," she thrust the coins in Max's hands. "Give them these."

Max flashed her a grin, shook himself free from Dad's grasp, and sprinted over to the musicians. When he came back, he stated happily, "That was five monies. That's a lot!"

Max threw his arms high in the air and sang, "*Life, I love you. All is funky!*" at the top of his lungs, while twirling around the platform. "*Hello, Subway, whatcha' doin'?*" Max continued, pausing to speak to the nearby pillar. Even the somber-suited men waiting by the wall had to smile at Max's version of the song.

Dad put out an arm to keep Max from tumbling onto the train rails and looked over Hannah's shoulder at the subway map. "Long way downtown," he observed.

Max put his solo on hold long enough to ask, "How many stops do we have to go?"

Just then a train roared into the station. They climbed on board, with Max insistent, "How many stops are we going to go, Daddy? How many? I want to know!"

As soon as they found a seat, Hannah put one finger on their stop at 77th Street and then pointed to the stop by Brooklyn Bridge. Max painstakingly counted, "One, two... thirteen!" he finally announced. "Thirteen stops! Wow!"

He tilted his head and looked up at Dad. "But, Daddy, our elevator skips thirteen. It goes eleven, twelve, fourteen. So does Kenny's. Maybe in New York we don't have thirteen anythings." Then Max corrected himself. "Except in school. In school we have to count thirteen—eleven, twelve, thirteen. So do we have thirteen stops or is it really fourteen?"

Dad rubbed his forehead. "Well, Buddy, it's only elevators that skip the number thirteen, not anything else. I don't know if it's just New York elevators or if elevators in other places do that, too."

"But why?" Max wanted to know.

"Because thirteen is an unlucky number," Hannah explained. "Nobody wants to live on the thirteenth floor of a building."

"I want to live on the thirteenth floor," Max announced. "When I grow up, I want my apartment to be on the thirteenth floor. Ok, Daddy?"

Dad raised his eyebrows and nodded.

In a minute, Max asked, "Why is thirteen unlucky?"

Hannah shrugged, so Dad answered, "There are lots of stories about why thirteen is considered unlucky, but they are just stories. There's even a word for being afraid of the number thirteen—*triskaidekaphobia*. I think it's a pretty silly thing to be afraid of!"

"Hannah," Max said, turning to face her. "Are you trisabia, kind of like you're afraid of escalators?"

"What?"

"You know, are you afraid of thirteen? You said you didn't want to live on the thirteenth floor in a building."

"No, I didn't. I meant people in general don't want to live on the thirteenth floor of a building. I don't know if I want to live on it or not."

Hannah looked up at Dad, who was holding on to the metal bar above their subway seats. Hannah thought out loud, "the thirteenth floor is still the thirteenth floor, even if they call it the fourteenth. You can't just change something's name and think that's going to make it different!"

Dad smiled and nodded in agreement.

Hannah looked at Max. "I'd live on the thirteenth floor. It wouldn't bother me. But I won't take an escalator to get up there!"

"Oh, goody," Max said. "We can have the same apartment when we're all growed up! On the thirteenth floor! That will be fun. And we will only take the elevator. I promise," he reassured Hannah with a pat on her knee.

Before she could protest this living arrangement, Dad ushered them off the train and on to the platform at Brooklyn Bridge.

Coming out of the station, their eyes had to adjust to the bright sunshine.

"Daddy," Max asked, "why are all these people here?" Max waved his hand in the direction of the bridge.

"I don't know, Buddy. It is certainly crowded, isn't it?" Dad turned to Hannah. "Which way now?"

Using the map, Hannah led them across the park in front of City Hall and through the maze of streets around the imposing building.

"Are we in a different city?" Max asked. "This doesn't look anything like where we live."

"Down here there aren't as many skyscrapers and the buildings are more massive. Also, streets don't make a neat grid like they do up in our neighborhood," Dad explained, showing Max the difference on the map. "So it feels like a different place."

"Mommy would get lost here," Max declared. Mom didn't have a very good sense of direction.

"Yeah, she probably would," Dad agreed.

"Look!" Hannah announced triumphantly. "There it is! Thomas Paine Park!"

They crossed the street into the park, and Hannah looked around slowly. "Is this all there is?" She was a little disappointed. "It's pretty small." It had taken how many months for her to finally get down here? And this little patch was all there was to Thomas Paine Park? It was mostly concrete!

Dad looked around carefully, too. "Well," he said finally, "at least there's a sign. It does have his name." The green sign proclaiming *Thomas Paine Park* was the same one with the maple leaf that marked all the parks run by the city government.

"You'd think, for someone as important to the Revolution as he was, there'd be a little more than just a sign," Dad said.

"And a bigger park," Hannah added.

"Where's the park?" Max asked. "I don't see any park. No playground." He waved his arms all around, looking fruitlessly for climbing equipment.

Dad laughed. "No playground here, that's for sure. It's a real city park, I guess."

Hannah's shoulders drooped. All that effort to get down here and this was it? And how did getting down here help their history project? Defeated, she was also a bit annoyed with Ms. Calde—what a dumb assignment! Thomas Paine deserved more than this little bit of Manhattan.

"Thirteen," she muttered to herself. "It was the thirteenth stop—how perfect. Maybe I *should* develop triskaideka-phobia."

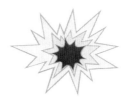

chapter 29
the brooklyn bridge

d addy, can we please walk over the Brooklyn Bridge? Please?" Max begged. The huge metal spider web arched into view as they rounded the corner near the subway stop.

Dad thought a minute. "I don't see why not. But there's not really anything on the other side, Buddy. Just so you know."

"Yes, there is," Max protested. "Brooklyn is on the other side!"

"True," Dad conceded, "but once we get to the other side, we still have to walk a ways for a snack..." Dad's voice trailed off as they were engulfed by a wide stream of people crossing the bridge. Dad immediately reached for Max's hand.

"Ronald McDonald House Fun Run," Hannah read the t-shirts passing by.

"I guess they're raising money for the Ronald McDonald House," Dad said.

"Ronald McDonald doesn't give out French fries at his house. I know because Mommy told me," Max said proudly.

"Hey, look!" Max said a moment later, pointing. "All those kids are baldies, just like Mommy."

"Max!" Hannah reminded him, exasperated.

"Oh, right, they're not baldies. They're just bald. But," Max turned to look Dad full on in the face, "that doesn't mean they have cankser."

"*Cancer*," Hannah hissed futilely under her breath.

"He's getting closer," Dad said, with a smile in Hannah's direction.

Then Dad nodded toward Max and acknowledged, "It's true, being bald doesn't mean you have cancer. But actually, these kids may have cancer. Kids with cancer often stay at the Ronald McDonald House with their families. The Ronald McDonald House in New York is just a few blocks from our apartment."

Hannah tried not to stare at the kids as they passed. Their shiny heads made them stand out, though, and it was hard not to look twice. One little boy, who was about Max's age, raised his arms up with a grin and careened wildly through the mass of people.

"*Life, I love you, all is groovy...,*'" Hannah hummed to herself, picturing Max's subway platform performance. "But," she paused suddenly in her thinking, "life isn't groovy for that kid. He has cancer."

Hannah turned to watch the group leave the bridge. The little boy continued spinning, twirling right into his mother's arms. She lifted him up, and they spun together, their whirling hug danced giggles up the bridge.

"They aren't baldies," Hannah whispered to herself. "They're people, just like Max and me."

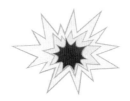

chapter 30
the beginning of the end

iz, we should do something to celebrate the end of your chemo," Dad said to Mom at dinner one night later that week.

Hannah glanced over at the calendar on the refrigerator. Was it already the middle of April?

"I know, just one more session," Mom said with a tired smile.

It would be great to see Mom in something besides her sweat suit. And earrings again. Mom didn't look like herself without earrings. Maybe a little makeup would be forthcoming, too? Hannah was cautiously optimistic.

"For you guys as well," Mom added. "You've practically been through chemo with me."

"Well, I haven't thrown up," Max said, gnawing on a pork chop.

"Thank goodness!" Mom said, turning a little green and putting down her fork.

"What should we do?" Dad persisted.

"Oh, I don't know. We should just be thankful it's over," Mom shrugged.

"Moooom!" Hannah groaned. "We have to do more than that! A party, maybe?" she suggested hopefully.

"No, no party." Mom shook her head. "Unless it's a thank you party for everyone who has helped out so much. I'm still too tired for a party."

"We could cook you a special dinner," Hannah offered.

Mom stared past Hannah at the wall. "I wish there was some way we could pass on all the help people have given us." She shook her head ruefully. "But right now I don't have any ideas or energy."

Dad's plate clattered on the kitchen counter. Max followed closely behind, licking his fingers and inquiring about dessert. "Let's clear the table first. Bring Mom's plate to the kitchen and then Hannah's." Dad directed. "Then we will talk dessert."

"Mom," Hannah began while the guys were in the kitchen. "Mom, we saw some kids with cancer doing a walk when we went to Thomas Paine Park."

Mom nodded. "I know. Max told me about them." She smiled. "He was very taken with the fact that chemo makes kids bald, too. He wanted to know if Matt was bald by now."

"Mom, could we do something for them? You know, since the Ronald McDonald House is so close to our apartment."

Mom pursed her lips and looked at Hannah. "What did you have in mind?"

"I don't know," Hannah admitted. "But somehow, seeing those kids out, trying to be normal people, even though right now, their lives are not normal at all…well, it just made me want to do something for them. But I don't know what."

Mom blinked slowly and rested her chin in her palm. "I think that's a great idea. Whenever I've seen sick children at the hospital or in the treatment rooms this year…" Mom shuddered. "I just don't know how they handle it. I've actually felt blessed that I was the one sick and not one of you. Let's think about what we can do."

Max waltzed into the dining area with a container of cookies. "Susan brought over chocolate chip cookies!" he announced, licking his lips. Hannah reached into the container eagerly. Susan's chocolate chip cookies were the best.

Mom waved the container away, crawled back on the sofa, and, despite the warmer weather, pulled the blanket up to her chin.

h annah," Mom said as Hannah came through the door the next afternoon. "I called the Ronald McDonald House today…"

Hannah shook her head on her way back to her room. "Not now, Mom. We have History Project presentations tomorrow and I've got to practice."

Hannah dropped her backpack on the floor, shut the door, cleared her throat, and began lecturing her stuffed animal about the American Revolution.

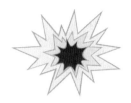

chapter 31
celebration time

h ow'd it go?" Mom asked anxiously the next afternoon
at pick-up time. She raised her hand, and a plastic
grocery bag dangled from her fingers. "I brought your
group a little treat."

Mary, Scottie, and Sam all crowded around eagerly.
Mom opened a box of tiny white cupcakes with toothpick flags
stuck in them. "Flags, for Betsy Ross and the Revolution, get
it?" Mom prompted.

The group grinned, and Hannah rolled her eyes. Max
crammed a cupcake in his mouth. "And for my birthday!" he
announced loudly. Max's birthday was on Flag Day, and he
always celebrated with a giant cake frosted to look like a flag.

"Max!" Mom said, exasperated. "Please show some
manners! And no, these are not for your birthday. These are in
honor of Hannah's group and what I am sure was a very
successful presentation."

Scottie looked at Mom mischievously. "But Liz, Betsy
Ross was in Philadelphia. I don't think we can eat those."

Sam mumbled through cupcake crumbs, "Well, these cupcakes are in New York. And they sure taste good!" He turned to Mom. "Thanks!"

Mary carefully took one from the plastic tray. "Did you make these?" she asked Mom politely.

Mom laughed. "Oh, no. I haven't cooked since last fall! There's a grocery store on the next block." She waved her hand in the direction of 79th Street. "This morning, I saw the flags at Rainbow…"

"The store that has everything!" Max interjected excitedly, spewing sugar everywhere.

Mom reached into her bag for a wipe for him and then repeated, "I saw the little flags at Rainbow, and I couldn't resist. They were so perfect for today." She offered the tray again to the group. "Here, have another one."

Hannah licked white frosting from her lips, relieved that the day was over.

"Well?" Mom asked again. "How'd it go?"

Scottie nodded. "We did OK," he allowed. He nodded his head slowly, the twitch of his lips belying his serious demeanor. "We did pretty good…"

"Just OK?" Sam stared at Scottie in disbelief. "No, not just OK. Not just pretty good. We did great! Really great! Magnificently, even!" Sam put up his hand for high fives and spun around. Hannah had never seen Sam this excited. Mom handed out more wipes.

Mary added, "Ms. Calde said that we addressed the stereotypes of the Revolution and where they came from particularly well. She thought it was especially interesting that we looked at the war from both sides."

Mom grinned, too, and high-fived them all.

Scottie said, "It was all Hannah's idea. We wouldn't have thought to organize it that way without Hannah's brainstorm, even if it did come a little late in the game."

"Yeah, I wasn't too happy about the change in our plan a couple of weeks ago," Sam allowed. "But it worked out super!" He reached for another cupcake. "And now I actually understand the Revolution a lot better. We're kind of lucky we're not still British!"

Scottie adopted a fake British accent and rested a make-believe silver tray on his fingertips. "Will you have some Earl Grey with your scones, My Lady?" He bowed low and offered a faux snack to Mom.

Mom tousled his hair with a smile. "Maybe that's why I like tea so much—perhaps I'm still a little bit British!"

As she was walking out of the schoolyard with Mom and Max, Hannah suddenly asked, "Mom, can Mary come over for a play date sometime soon?"

"Sure," Mom said brightly, for the first time in a long time. "My last treatment is on Thursday. I won't feel good for about a week, but then we'll get her over. You guys talk about it at school, and I'll give her mom a call."

Hannah grinned. *Sure* was a word she liked to hear, and it was so good to be talking about the future.

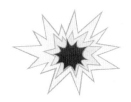

chapter 32
game time planning

"We're going to go and just play games," Hannah told Mary over apples and caramel dip at the dining room table.

"That sounds like fun," Mary said. "Do you know what games?"

"The lady Mom spoke to wanted to make sure we were willing to play Uno. She said that one little boy in particular really liked that game and that his mom never wanted to see a deck of Uno cards again!" Hannah grinned. "That's not a problem. Even Max can play Uno!"

"You know who likes Uno?" Mary said thoughtfully. "Sam. He loves it and he actually has all these strategies for winning."

"Strategies?" Hannah shook her head in disbelief. "Strategies for winning Uno? There's no such thing!"

"I don't know," Mary shrugged. "You'll have to ask him."

"When we had the idea, Mom called the Ronald McDonald House to see how we could help. They didn't really have anything specific they needed done, but t They said what the kids most needed was to feel normal. So Mom said she could so relate to that. Mom and I were trying hard to think of something normal that most of the kids at the Ronald McDonald House would feel like doing. That's how we came up with a game afternoon.

"The lady was also a little worried that we might be upset because they were bald. But, I guess it helps that I'm so used to seeing Mom without a hat. I don't think seeing anyone else with a bald head will bother me."

Hannah continued, bubbling over with excitement for their project. "Max thought we should bring pizza…"

"No, I didn't!" Max drove his truck by the table to grab an apple slice. "I wanted them to have French fries!" He leveled his gaze intently at Mary. "When Mommy was sick, French fries would have made her feel better." Then he sighed dramatically, "But Ronald McDonald doesn't have French fries at his house."

Mary held the bowl of caramel down for him. Max made a face, "Yuck!" and steered himself out through the kitchen.

"…but," Hannah picked right back up, "Mom said that she didn't know how pizza would sit with their stomachs and all the various treatments. So we're just going to play games. Dad says he hopes someone will be up for a good game of Monopoly!"

Hannah giggled. "I hope they're ready to hand over all their money. Dad likes to win!"

"I'm bringing my trains!" Max announced, bringing a truckload of tracks into the dining area. "Hannah, do you think someone will play trains with me there?"

Mary reassured him. "The boys there will be very impressed by all of your trains. You can show them how to build a really complicated track."

Max dumped his load and drove back towards the bedroom.

Mary turned to Hannah. "This sounds like a really fun afternoon. Do you think I could come, too? I like to play games, and I don't think bald heads would bother me."

"Sure!" Hannah enthused. "I'm sure you can. I mean...I'll have to ask Mom." Then she grinned a little mischievously. " I know how we can find out if baldness is an issue for you."

Before Mary could reply, Hannah turned her head towards the kitchen and yelled in a panicked voice, "Mom, can you come here? We need help!"

Mom came running in, bareheaded. "What is it? If everything OK?" she wanted to know, alarmed.

Hannah eyed Mary looking at Mom. "Nope, you'll be fine," she pronounced.

Mary flushed and Mom looked confused.

"We were just finding out whether bald heads would bother Mary if she came to help at the Ronald McDonald House." Hannah explained to Mom. Then she added, "She doesn't seem fazed by yours."

Mom covered her head involuntarily with her hands and turned a little pink. "So there's nothing wrong?"

When Hannah shook her head, Mom rolled her eyes. "Hannah! You know not to cry wolf. That's never a good..."

"I know, I know," Hannah waved Mom off. "But it worked, and now we know that Mary's not bothered by bald heads."

Mom left the room to get her hat, and Hannah turned back to Mary. "Hey, do you think Scottie and Sam might want to come too?"

Mary nodded slowly. "Yeah, I'm pretty sure they would. Sam loves to play *Uno* and Scottie can make anyone laugh."

Max drove another load of train tracks into the dining area and dumped them. Mary licked the caramel off her fingers and squatted down to help him hold the bridge steady. "You know, Lydia can do manicures," she said thoughtfully.

Hannah clinked the dishes into the sink. "She's never painted my fingernails. Has she done yours?" Hannah asked curiously. She didn't think Mary and Lydia were that close.

Mary shook her head. "No, but some of the girls at the Ronald McDonald House might like to have a manicure."

Mom walked into the dining area with her baseball cap back on and carrying a cup of tea in her hands. At the word *manicure*, she glanced at her own hands ruefully. Chemo had made her nails really soft, so she kept them really short and ignored them as much as possible.

"Oh, no!" Hannah shook her head vigorously. "No way is Lydia coming. She'd just try to be in charge of everything."

"Maybe not, if you already have a plan in place and tell her what her part is," Mom interrupted. "I think she'd like to be included. And I'm pretty sure some of those kids would love to have their nails done.

"It's a good idea," Mom said to Mary, "to include Lydia, but to give her a very specific part to do. She *is* bossy," Mom

202

nodded in agreement with Hannah, "but I think she does want to be part of the group. If she knows she's being included and what her role is, then I bet you some of her bossiness will evaporate."

Hannah fell off her chair in mock horror. "Lydia's bossiness evaporate? Dost thou know what thou sayest?! Impossible!"

Mary giggled as Max returned with some of his trains to try out on the track. "You've been hanging around Scottie too much," Mary told Hannah.

After a minute, Hannah said, "Besides, Lydia would probably make some mean comment about them not having any hair."

"Wait a minute," Mom said. "Why couldn't we do to Lydia what you just did to Mary?"

"What?" Hannah asked.

"Why couldn't we show Lydia my bald head and see what her reaction is. Maybe if she saw my head out there shining in all its bald glory a few times, then other bald heads wouldn't bother her."

"Oh, no!" Hannah's eyes widened in alarm. "You are not showing your head to Lydia!"

"Why not? You just had me show it to Mary," Mom retorted.

"But that was different..."

Mom raised her eyebrows.

"It was!" Hannah insisted.

Mom smiled. "Well, it's something to think about, anyway." She picked up her mug and walked over to the telephone.

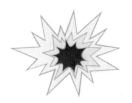

chapter 33
party time!

hannah squirmed under the covers as she heard Mom's off-key singing, "…*so rise and shine and give God the glory, glory. Rise and shine and…*" Light slithered through the opening in the blinds, driving Hannah to bury her head further under the pillow.

"Enough already!" Hannah muttered.

Mom must have had success in rousing Max because her tune faded out into the hallway.

A few minutes later, a hand rubbed Hannah's back through the covers. "Come on, Sleepyhead," Dad cautioned sympathetically, "or Mom will come in and sing some more…"

Hannah sighed and worked her way down to the ladder at the end of her bed. The fact that Mom's energy was coming back wasn't always a good thing.

Once they were all at the table eating breakfast, Dad asked, "So what's on the agenda today?"

"Today's my art day," Max announced happily. "I looooove art!"

Mom eyed his shirt over a spoonful of raisin bran. "Perhaps we should change your shirt, M.D.. White is not a good color for you on art days."

Max looked down at his clothes. "Nooooooo, don't make me change! I like this shirt, Mommy. It's my dino shirt! And it's short-sleeved! I loooooovvvvvveee short-sleeved shirts. They let my arms be free! Please, don't make me change…"

Dad pointed to Max's oatmeal and pantomimed eating. When Max opened his mouth to protest some more, Dad shoveled in a real bite. Then Dad looked at Hannah, "And you?"

"Um, well," Hannah said as she bit off the tip of her banana. She swallowed. "Ms. Calde said we're having a special guest today. But she wouldn't say any more. I think the person's coming after lunch. Other than that, it's just a regular day."

Nodding at her, Dad next turned to Mom. "I've got a trip I need to make soon for work, but I've got a little flexibility around when it happens. Is it OK if I give you a call from the office? Then we can compare calendars from there."

Mom nodded. "Anytime before 2:00 is fine. I'll be here—today is paperwork day." She waved her hand in the direction of the computer desk. A pile of bills stood ready and waiting.

a t 2:10, Ms. Calde lined the class up.
"Where are we going?" Carl asked. "Aren't we supposed to have a special guest this afternoon anyway?"

Ms. Calde smiled mysteriously and brought the line into the hallway. Lydia led the way downstairs, swishing her ponytail dramatically behind her. Scottie caught Hannah's eye and shrugged. Mary and Sam faced forward, as usual following directions meticulously.

205

At the bottom of the stairs in the lunchroom, Lydia paused, looking around for some evidence of the mystery guest.

"Lydia, this way," Ms. Calde gestured. She opened the door into the schoolyard. The line filed through the door to the outside. In the corner a table was layered with balloons. In the middle of all the color sat what looked like an enormous cake.

Just as Ms. Calde indicated they should keep walking towards the table, Max tore through the lunchroom and out the door. "Hannah! Hannah! It's a party!" he shouted over his shoulder.

Mom followed closely behind him, and behind her were Ellie, Ken, Lucy, Ryan, Robert, and Ian.

"Max? Mom?" Hannah wondered questioningly. Mom smiled at Hannah and then looked past her at the outside gate.

Mom's smile split into a grin upon seeing a tall man in a business suit opening the gate and letting himself in. "John!" She waved him over.

"Dad?" Hannah stammered. What was going on?

"Daddy!" Max shrieked joyfully. He ran over to the gate and leapt into Dad's arms.

"Why is your whole family here?" Lydia turned to Hannah.

"I have no idea," Hannah replied shaking her head. "No idea whatsoever."

"Looks like a party to me," Scottie said, strolling towards the table in the back. "Yep, it's a cake. Wanna come read it, Hannah?"

All of Hannah's classmates, plus the other friends Mom had collected, gathered around the table. Carl pushed his arms into the crowd. "Let the lady through. Clear a path and let the lady through," he sang.

Hannah walked the aisle Carl had created, completely confused. When she got to the front, Scottie grinned at her and pointed to the cake.

"Towards A New Normal...An End of Chemo Celebration!" was written in bright pink frosting on top of the biggest cake Hannah had ever seen. She looked up at Mom.

"It's the party you wanted me to have...the End of Chemo Party," Mom said. "But it's not just for me. It's for all of us." Then she turned to all the kids and took off her baseball cap. Hannah blushed as most of the kids stared.

"I sure am glad it's warming up! Now I won't have to wear my hat all the time," Mom began. The quiet was deafening.

Mom continued, "I don't know how many of you know that our family has been dealing with cancer this year. It's been a bit of a challenging year. The good news is I finished chemo about a month ago, and even better, my hair is starting to grow back." Hannah watched the kids squint, looking hard at Mom's head. Unless you were up very close, you couldn't see her fuzz. It was coming back really light-colored, maybe even, Mom worried, gray.

Mom addressed the group some more, "But I appreciate how much all of you have helped us, even if you didn't know it. You've been Hannah and Max's friends, and that's the best thing in the whole world you could have done.

"Hannah was very disappointed when I didn't have an end-of-chemo party a little while ago." Mom smiled over all the heads at Hannah. "She is wonderful enough to think that that was worth a celebration."

"Mommy," Max interrupted, standing on his tiptoes, "when we have the cake, can I please have a rose?" He leaned over to Kenny and whispered loudly, " I like to lick the frosting part off. But I never eat the cake. It's yucky."

The grownups laughed. Mom wiped her cheek quickly with her fingertips. "Oh, before I get mushy...we wanted Hannah and Max to get to celebrate with all their friends and we wanted to thank you all for being great kids."

Dad handed the knife over the crowd to Mom and she made the first cut.

"No more chemo!" Scottie cheered, and the rest of the kids began to chant, "No more chemo! No more chemo!" until everyone had a slice of cake. Then there was silence, broken only by the smacking of more than a few lips.

Dad pulled an iPod and some speakers from his pocket. After he pushed a few buttons, everyone started bobbing to *It's the End of the World as We Know It.*"

"My dad loves this song!" Sam said, doing a fancy dance step. Hannah couldn't believe her eyes. This was twice now in the past month Sam had surprised her.

thank you, Liz. The cake was delicious," Mary said as Ms. Calde rounded up the class to start upstairs.

"Yeah! Thanks, Liz! Awesome surprise!" Scottie seconded. "By the way, the hairstyle is extremely flattering. Buzz cuts are really in right now, you know."

Mom rolled her eyes and chuckled, shaking her head. "Glad you like it, Scottie. You know how worried I am about being fashion-forward!"

Scottie flashed a peace sign to her on his way to line up.

"I'm sorry you were sick," Sam said. "But I'm glad you're feeling better now. That cake was awfully good." Mom smiled at him.

Mrs. Calde beckoned to the kids Mom had corralled to come who were not in her class. "You need to go up with us. It's nearly dismissal time."

Ellie and Lucy gave Mom quick hugs. Mom dabbed at her eyes again. Then she grabbed Kenny, Ryan, and Ian who were running laps in the yard with Max. "Go on up with Ms. Calde. She'll get you to your teacher. It's almost time to go home."

Suddenly, the schoolyard was empty except for the Bennetts. Mom bent over to pick up a paper plate.

Hannah slid her arms around Mom's waist. "Thank you, Mom," she whispered.

Mom twisted around and righted herself in Hannah's hug. "No, thank you, Sweetie. You and Max got me through this. I don't know what I would have done without you."

Hannah buried her head in Mom's clothes, and they stood there until Max crawled in under their legs and poked his head up between their bellies. He grinned. "I love parties!"

"Hey," Dad protested from where he was cleaning up on the other side of the yard. "If it's a family hug, then I need to be in on it, too." He walked over and encircled all three of them with his long arms.

After a minute, Hannah squirmed out. "OK, enough. School's almost out and very soon there are going to be a bunch of kids out here."

"Go get your backpack," Mom told her. "I'll take Max up to his room."

"So that was a little embarrassing," Hannah said as she packed up her bag in the classroom.

"Why? It was a great party!" Carl threw his reading book onto his pile of stuff.

"Well, she didn't have to take off her hat…" Hannah murmured.

"Why not?" Scottie asked, picking up his clarinet case. "It's kind of like a badge of honor."

"But not in front of everyone," Hannah protested.

"We don't care," Mary told her, walking over to the closet.

As the rest of the class collected their belongings and headed out the door, Lydia lingered over her zipper much longer than usual. Just as Hannah fastened her last strap, Lydia lifted her head and looked at Hannah.

"I'm really sorry about your mom. I know you told me and everything, but," Lydia shrugged, "I guess until I saw her head, I didn't believe it."

"Yeah," Hannah said. "Baldness kind of yells 'cansker'…"

Lydia raised her eyebrows.

"Uh," Hannah blushed. Had she really just used a Maxism? Hannah cleared her throat. "Cancer. Baldness yells *cancer*."

Then Hannah added, "But don't feel sorry for her. That's the last thing Mom wants."

"And I'm sorry I bugged you about play dates," Lydia continued, averting her gaze.

"I probably should have told you sooner," Hannah conceded. "But I just didn't want everyone to know."

As they started down the steps, Lydia changed the subject. "Hey, I heard Mary and Scottie talking about some project you guys are doing."

"You did?" Hannah replied weakly.

"Yeah, something about playing games with some kids on a Saturday afternoon...I'm really good at games. Why don't I plan on giving lessons on how to play Menkala? It's my favorite game in the whole world! Just so I can check my calendar, when you going?"

As an afterthought, Lydia added, "And where?"

Hannah sighed. There was no reforming Lydia. She would always be bossy. Then Hannah saw Mary wave up to her from the foot of the stairs.

Hannah smiled and waved back. She put her arm around Lydia's shoulders as they started down the stairs. "You know, Lydia, I think we've got the games all covered. But you'd be really great at giving manicures. We don't have anybody to do that..."

Someone shoved the door to the schoolyard open, and she and Lydia went, arm in arm, to join the rest of their class in the bright sunshine.

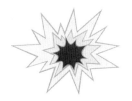

acknowledgments

I would like to thank Kira Henschel at HenschelHaus Publishing for her willingness to publish this book from an unknown author.

I appreciate the care I received at Memorial Sloan-Kettering Cancer Center after my diagnosis of breast cancer. Drs. Alexandra Heerdt, Andrew Seidman, and Peter Cordeira, and their staffs, followed me through and healed me from a scary time. Their continued care through my regular check-ups and periodic panics is much appreciated.

I would like to thank Dr. Seidman in particular for commenting on portions of this manuscript. I really appreciate his taking the time out of his very busy schedule to do so, as well as his enthusiasm for the project.

I can't thank my friends and family enough. People supported us from the moment I had a suspicious mammogram. I love and appreciate beyond measure: my parents, Jo Ann and Joe Morrison; my in-laws, Jean Friedman and Bernard Dauenhauer, and my late mother-in-law Mary Dauenhauer; my sisters and their spouses, Ashley and Adam Robertson, Whitney and Bob Saunders; my brother-in-law and sister-in-law and their family, Christine and David Dauenhauer, Peter,

Jack, and Patrick; my aunt and uncle, Lamar and Doug Webb; their children and spouses, Annie and Doug Webb, Marcy Webb and Matt Reid, and Kat and Charlie Webb-Whedbee.

I know I'll omit someone with a list of friends! But in an effort to say a heartfelt thank you, here goes: Kathleen, Todd, Michelle, Steve, Laurie, Nina, Karyn, Stephanie, Caroline, Nevin, Deb, Patty, Georgia, Brad, Melissa, Lallande, Greg, Zorina, Raegan, Robert, Katherine, Suzanne, Chris, Mike, Christina, Lori, Sidney, Tina, Mary, Caroline, Carissa, Maureen, Anne, Marianne, Alyssa, Anne, Jackie, Jennifer, Anna, Michelle, Ginger, Carole, Lisa, and Leslie. The meals, laundry, ironing, play dates, cards, moral support, and prayers were the only way we got through.

That list doesn't mention the wonderful new friends I've made since we moved from New York. Their kindness and interest have been a major source of support (and kick in the pants) during the publication process. In particular, Jan and the Christ Renews group, you've been a real godsend. And Tina, you can proofread my stuff anytime!

Above all, I want to acknowledge my family: I am grateful every day that my husband Mark Dauenhauer asked me to marry him. That I've discovered his editing abilities is an added bonus. My children, Madeleine and Joseph Dauenhauer, are the reason I get up in the morning. I am so excited to see what wonderful things they do with their lives!

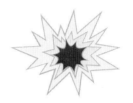

About the Author

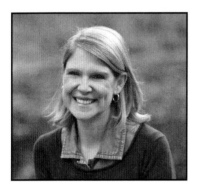

ansley M. Dauenhauer is a former elementary school teacher and science museum coordinator/educator. She has published several magazine and newspaper articles and essays. *Cancer Slam* is her first novel.

She and her husband Mark have lived in both New York City and London, as well as up and down the East Coast. They recently relocated to Michigan with their two children, Maddie and Joseph, where they enjoy reading, camping, hiking, exploring new places, and hanging out at home.

Please visit her at www.ansleymdauenhauer.com.

Three Towers Press is a division of HenschelHAUS Publishing, Inc.
We are happy to review manuscripts from new and veteran authors
and offer a wide range of author services,
such as coaching, editing, design, and book marketing.

Please visit www.HenschelHAUSBooks.com for submission guidelines,
our on-line bookstore, and calendar of workshops and author events.